# THE ROLE OF
# DIAGNOSIS
# IN PSYCHIATRY

# THE ROLE OF
# DIAGNOSIS
# IN PSYCHIATRY

## R. E. KENDELL

M.D., F.R.C.P., M.R.C. Psych.
Professor of Psychiatry
University of Edinburgh

**BLACKWELL SCIENTIFIC PUBLICATIONS**

OXFORD LONDON EDINBURGH MELBOURNE

© 1975 Blackwell Scientific Publications
Osney Mead, Oxford,
85 Marylebone High Street, London W1,
9 Forrest Road, Edinburgh,
P.O. Box 9, North Balwyn, Victoria, Australia.

ISBN 0 632 00701 X

First published 1975

Distributed in the United States of America by
J. B. Lippincott Company, Philadelphia and in
Canada by J. B. Lippincott Company Ltd.,
Toronto
Printed and bound in Great Britain by
Aberdeen University Press

# Contents

# Contents

# Preface

Eighty years ago Hack Tuke observed that 'The wit of man has rarely been more exercised than in the attempt to classify the morbid mental phenomena covered by the term insanity', and went on to add that the result had been disappointing. The remark remains as apposite now as it was then, and goes far towards explaining why many present day psychiatrists have lost interest in the whole issue of diagnosis, while others have suggested that it is an unnecessary, even a harmful exercise. This book was born of the conviction that such attitudes are profoundly mistaken, and that the development of a reliable and valid classification of the phenomena of mental illness, and of the unambiguous diagnostic criteria which are essential to this task, are two of the most important problems facing contemporary psychiatry. Certainly the failure of both psychiatrists and psychologists to develop a satisfactory classification of their subject matter, or even to agree on the principles on which that classification should be based, is a most serious barrier to fruitful research into the aetiology of mental illness and even into the efficacy of therapeutic regimes. It is more exciting to develop explanatory theories, or to claim impressive results for this or that treatment, than it is to define the critical characteristics of the patients on whom one's research was based. It is probably more exciting to an architect to design parabolic canopies or baroque façades than it is to calculate the size and shape of the concrete slab on which his building will rest. But theories and therapeutic claims have no more chance of surviving than buildings if they are not built on secure foundations. Developing reliable diagnostic criteria and a valid classification may be as tedious as filling muddy holes with concrete but both provide the foundations on which all else depends.

It is not my purpose here to advocate any particular solution to the diagnostic controversies which have plagued psychiatry for so long, or to present a novel classification of my own. Part of the problem is that too many people have done this already. I have tried rather to discuss and clarify some of the conceptual and semantic problems involved, to explain why it has been so difficult to achieve adequate reliability, or even agreement on a common nomenclature, and to set out the principles that should govern attempts to resolve these problems in the future. If we are to avoid repeating the mistakes of the past and a further cycle of failure and disappointment we must decide what we mean by terms like 'disease' and 'entity'; we must appreciate what diagnoses are, why they are necessary, and also what distortions they impose on our thinking; above all we must realize the importance of unambiguous operational or semantic definitions for all our diagnostic labels. We must also have some understanding of the perceptual and cognitive processes involved in the act of making a diagnosis; and if we are to make a rational choice between categorical and dimensional classifications, and appreciate the ways in which computers can and cannot help us, we must try to understand the various forms of multivariate analysis that have been applied to classificatory problems, and their many limitations.

Although this book is primarily an attempt to further these aims, it may also serve to illustrate the contemporary medical concept of mental illness to members of other professional groups. At all events, the assumptions made by behavioural scientists, and popular writers like Szasz and Laing, about what they call the 'medical model' have sometimes been inaccurate or outdated, and their arguments might carry greater conviction if they had a better understanding of the concepts they are criticizing, and the factual basis from which they are derived. Important as such misconceptions are, this book is aimed mainly at those directly concerned with the study and treatment of mental illness, and its central purpose is to remind them that diagnosis and classification are matters of fundamental importance, and to stimulate them to think about, and act on, the themes that are developed in the following pages.

Few books are ever written by their authors alone, and I cannot omit to record my gratitude to several of my colleagues in the preparation and revision of this one. In particular I would like to thank Sir Denis Hill, Professor A. E. Maxwell and Dr Norman Sartorius for their detailed and invaluable comments on the chapters in which I was really straying into the territory of their expertise, and Dr Norman Kreitman for his careful appraisal of the final manuscript. Above all, I am grateful to my secretary Liz Boxley for her efficiency, enthusiasm and patience.

R.E.K.
The Institute of Psychiatry
March 1974

# 1 The Importance of Diagnosis

In most branches of medicine the value of diagnosis is never questioned. Its importance is self-evident because treatment and prognosis are largely determined by it. If a man of forty with a cough and bloodstained sputum is diagnosed as having pulmonary tuberculosis, it follows almost automatically that he will be treated with isoniazid for several months, probably in combination with other anti-tuberculous drugs, and at the end of that time his health is likely to be restored. If, on the other hand, he is diagnosed as having a bronchial carcinoma his treatment and prognosis will both be quite different. He may have a pneumonectomy or radiotherapy, or neither, but either way he will not receive isoniazid. If he is fortunate his health may be restored, but it is much more likely that he will be dead within two years, and, depending on the site and extent of his disease, a fairly accurate estimate can be made of his chances of survival. It is also unlikely that there will be any disagreement about the diagnosis. The history and findings on physical examination may be equivocal, and the initial impressions of different doctors may conflict with one another. However, after a few days of investigations, chest X Ray, bronchoscopy, sputum examination and so on, the diagnosis will usually be beyond dispute, even if the patient has both illnesses.

Where mental illness is concerned the situation is rather different. A man of forty who is sleeping badly, cannot think clearly and suspects that his colleagues are talking about him behind his back may have either schizophrenia or a depressive illness. If he is schizophrenic, he is likely to be treated with phenothiazines, and to recover incompletely, or become chronically ill. If he has a depressive illness, he is more likely to be treated with ECT or a tricyclic antidepressant, and to recover completely within two or three months. But whichever diagnosis he is given, he may still receive phenothiazines, or ECT, or a tricyclic drug, or even all three, and may recover completely, incompletely, or not at all. Psychiatrists are quite likely to disagree amongst themselves whether he has schizophrenia or an affective illness, and even about the definition and meaning of these two terms. They may even make a diagnosis of 'schizoaffective illness',

1

which to many clinicians must seem tantamount to making a diagnosis of 'tuberculoplasm' in a patient who has some symptoms suggesting that he has tuberculosis and others suggesting that he has a neoplasm.

This is the fundamental reason why the importance of diagnosis is not self-evident in psychiatry in the way that it is in other branches of medicine; because the therapeutic and prognostic implications of psychiatric diagnoses are relatively weak, and the diagnoses themselves relatively unreliable. Psychiatrists tend to react to this state of affairs in one of three ways. Those who are most strongly influenced by medical tradition usually minimize or deny the problem, insisting that diagnosis is crucial to rational treatment and sometimes striving to demonstrate clear relationships between diagnosis and therapeutic response. The majority admit the problem and react by taking less and less interest in the whole question of diagnosis. They continue, out of habit, to assign diagnoses to their patients, but the criteria they use become blunt and vague through neglect, and they are not disturbed when their colleagues' diagnoses differ from their own because they regard it as an 'academic matter' without any practical importance. As a result, diagnostic reliability falls further and a vicious circle develops as therapeutic and prognostic implications become even more tenuous and uncertain. A third group, people like Neumann in the last century and Karl Menninger in this, advocate abandoning diagnosis outright and argue persuasively the advantages, even the necessity, of doing so.

THE SHORTCOMINGS OF DIAGNOSES

There are indeed many problems and pitfalls associated with the act of assigning a diagnosis to a 'dis-eased' human being, particularly where psychiatry is concerned, and it may be as well to recognize these at the outset. In the first place, there are many situations in which a diagnosis seems almost pathetically inadequate to convey what we feel to be the essence of the patient's predicament. Karl Menninger, the most vocal and influential of contemporary abolitionists, has expressed the feeling very clearly (Menninger, 1948):

'What shall we call the "disease" represented by a man who has always been frail but has worked hard to support his widowed mother, did not feel he could afford to get married, buries himself in the details of a complicated job, develops paralysing headaches, loses time at the office for which pay is deducted from his wages, worries about this so much that he loses sleep and begins vomiting after each meal? Just to make it complicated he has a leukocytosis and an enlarged spleen. Does not such a disease defy diagnosis?'

'Even in the simplest cases it seems to me misleading to make a diagnosis in the old-fashioned way. A middle-aged puritan spinster appears in my office with a chancre on her lip. Isn't this a simple diagnosis? I don't think so. Nor would you if I told you the circumstances of how she acquired that chancre, whom she acquired it from, how she happened to select that type of man, or why she permitted him to kiss her. Her sickness cannot be accurately diagnosed just as syphilis. She did not come to me because of it. What she came to me for was a more serious thing. She was so depressed about the implications of the infection that she now wanted to kill herself. What is the name of that disease? . . . What is the diagnosis in a patient who has coronary symptoms whenever he takes his wife to a party? Or in a woman who has migraine on the weekends that her son is home from college? What kind of arthritis is it which becomes activated with each quarterly meeting of the board of directors?'

Not only does a formal diagnosis often fail to convey what we feel to be the essential elements of the problem, it may not even tell us what the patient's symptoms are, or how he came to medical attention, or how he should be treated, or even what is likely to happen to him without treatment. To be told that a patient has an anxiety neurosis, for instance, does not tell us why he is frightened, or why he consulted a doctor, whether he is tense all the time or terrified episodically, whether drugs, interpretive psychotherapy or any of numerous forms of behavioural treatment are likely to help him, how badly disabled he is, or whether he is likely to recover without treatment. A related problem is that the majority of patients do not conform to the tidy stereotyped descriptions found in textbooks. They possess some, but not all, of the symptoms of two or three different diagnostic categories and so have to be allocated more or less arbitrarily to whichever syndrome they most nearly resemble. As a result disagreements about diagnosis are frequent and patients' diagnoses change repeatedly as they move from one doctor or hospital to another.

THE HARMFUL EFFECTS OF DIAGNOSES

There are other equally important, if less tangible, objections to diagnoses, as Menninger has emphasized. Attaching a name to a condition creates a spurious impression of understanding so that we cease to be puzzled and to ask questions. To say that someone has schizophrenia really says little more than that he is behaving in a rather odd way which we have encountered in other people in the past, but to the layman, and to some doctors also, it implies that we understand what is wrong with him, that he has an 'illness' like measles or appendicitis whose cause we either know already or will soon discover, and that there is a fundamental difference between this and other kinds of odd behaviour. Hardin (1956) coined the word panchreston (meaning 'explain-all', by analogy with panacea, or 'cure-all') to draw attention to the ways in which we use our jargon to provide comforting but meaningless explanations for things we really do not understand. He did us a valuable service by doing so, but there may be other dimensions to the problem as well. It is worth recalling that the belief that names are invested with magical powers was once widespread amongst our ancestors. There are many surviving accounts and legends of kings and gods having special names known only to themselves and their most devoted followers and, as the stories of Aladdin and Rumplestiltskin illustrate, it was believed that anyone discovering the secret name thereby achieved power over its owner. It is perhaps not too fanciful to suggest that the lingering shadow of this belief is part of the reason why doctors and patients alike find it so comforting to have impressive Greek or Latin names for the sicknesses that oppress them. Doubtless there are also more mundane reasons why doctors choose to conceal their ignorance from their patients and their relatives by clothing it in a Greek neologism, but all too often they also deceive themselves and treat the disease instead of the patient.

This last effect, the subtle way in which making a diagnosis distracts the doctor from his primary function of trying to relieve the suffering of a 'dis-eased' person and encourages him to treat an inanimate disease instead, is the most important drawback of all in the eyes of many psychiatrists. They feel, with some justification, that, whatever other branches of medicine may do, psychiatry must be concerned with the patient as a person, including his hopes and fears, his memories and daydreams, and that to attribute a diagnosis to him is inevitably to dehumanize him and to deflect attention from him onto his biochemistry or his genes or his delusions. Like Adolph Meyer (1907), they insist that psychiatrists should be concerned with understanding the sick person in terms of his life experience rather than with fitting his symptoms into a classificatory scheme. Others go further, maintaining that it is demeaning to any human being to be labelled like a specimen in a museum. Although it may be a little fanciful to claim that all labelling is necessarily derogatory it is certainly true, as Albee (1970) and others have pointed out, that the act of assigning a diagnosis to a patient inevitably focuses attention on his deficiencies rather than on his assets, and also that many psychiatric diagnoses have strong pejorative connotations. It is by no means rare for the aura surrounding such terms as hysteric, neurotic, psychopath and schizophrenic to have harmful effects on people's behaviour and attitudes towards the patient so labelled, and on his own attitude to himself; and at times they are used, by professional personnel as well as by laymen, as little more than thinly disguised expressions of contempt. What is more, labels like schizophrenia are sometimes attached to people on wholly inadequate evidence, and once attached may be almost impossible to remove (Rosenhan, 1973).

THE CALL FOR THE ABANDONMENT OF DIAGNOSIS

In the face of this impressive catalogue of shortcomings, misuses and pitfalls it is hardly surprising that some critics have advocated doing away with diagnoses completely. In Menninger's words: 'We affirm the necessity of cutting the Gordian Knot and using no names at all for these conditions of mental illness' (Menninger, 1963). Instead, he and other psychoanalysts would substitute a lengthy formulation of each patient's predicament, describing his symptoms and their evolution, the strengths and weaknesses of his character, the nature of his relationships with other people, the stresses he was under and the way in which these played on his weaknesses and reopened old wounds, and the way in which his current behaviour and attitudes represent an attempt to defend himself against internal stresses. Every such formulation would be different, just as every human being is different, and would incorporate a plan of treatment tailored to the needs of that unique individual. (In fact, Menninger and many other psychiatrists still refer to this as a diagnosis; the term formulation is used here instead to avoid the ambiguity which would be bound to arise if the same word was used for the traditional label and for this comprehensive assessment.)

Essentially, Menninger's argument is that, because in one sense all mental illness rests on a single common foundation shared by all mankind, while in another equally important sense every individual is unique, and unique in his sickness, it is useless to classify either patients or illnesses; the sick individual must be assessed and treated on his own merits free from the pernicious restraints imposed by disease categories.

## The fallacy in the argument

This argument is based on a serious fallacy, which soon becomes apparent if we consider the functions of classification and class membership. Whatever the context, whether one is concerned with sickness or not, there are three aspects to every human being:
1. those he shares with all mankind
2. those he shares with some other men, but not all
3. those which are unique to him.
The value of classification in any given context depends on the size of the second of these categories relative to the other two. The larger the first category the less the need for classification, and the larger the third the less the value of any classification that is attempted. Implicit in Menninger's viewpoint is the assumption that where mental illness is concerned, the first and third of these categories overshadow the second, and that the second can therefore be ignored.

Let us take this assumption at face value to see where it leads. In so far as all men are the same we cannot distinguish between one type of mentally ill person and another. Indeed, we cannot even distinguish between those who are ill and those who are healthy. It follows from this that if we have more than one form of treatment at our disposal we can have no rational criteria for employing treatment A in one situation and treatment B in another. We cannot even discriminate between those who need treatment and those who do not. On the other hand, in so far as every individual is unique, all learning from experience and all useful communication with others are rendered impossible. If every patient is different from every other then we can learn nothing from our colleagues, our textbooks, or the accumulated experience of our predecessors. We cannot even learn from our own personal experience if there are no significant similarities between our last patient and the next. We may increase in skill and understanding in the course of treating one individual, but that skill and understanding will not carry over to the next. In short, insistence on a unitary concept of mental illness condemns us to giving the same treatment to every one, and prevents us even distinguishing between sickness and health. Insistence on the uniqueness of every individual prevents all learning and all communication concerning disease.

In fact, it is impossible to avoid classifying patients unless one is prepared to accept the facile Rogerian dictum that 'Therapy is good for people. Period.' and to offer the same panacea to everyone. As soon as one begins to recognize features that are common to some patients but not to all, and to distinguish those which are important from those, like eye colour, which are not, one is classifying them, whether one recognizes it or not. The only point at issue is what sort of classification one is going to have. As Pasamanick (1963) has pointed out, even our language is based on classification; every common noun expresses the recognition of a class. Menninger may well be correct in maintaining that, in comparison with physical illness, category (2) above is small where mental illness is concerned relative to categories (1) and (3), but we still have to focus our attention on category (2) if we are ever to acquire any useful understanding and pass that understanding on to others.

THE UNAVOIDABILITY OF DIAGNOSIS

In fact, the detailed personal formulation advocated as an alternative to a diagnosis is no alternative at all. The two are required for quite different purposes, and have different functions. A formulation which takes into account the unique features of the patient and his environment and the interaction between the two is often essential for any real understanding of his predicament, and for planning effective treatment, but it is unusable in any situation in which populations or groups of patients need to be considered. In any such situation some form of classification or categorization is unavoidable. It is important not to see this issue simply as a controversy between psychoanalysts and 'organic' psychiatrists. Feinstein and Kline, starting from quite different theoretical positions from Menninger, have also commented forcibly on the shortcomings of diagnoses in isolation, and argued convincingly that they need to be augmented by other data for research purposes just as much as in the management of the individual patient (Kline, Tenney, Nicolaou and Malzberg, 1953; Feinstein, 1964). But it is one thing to supplement a diagnosis with other information and quite another to abandon it. Without diagnosis, or some comparable method of classification, epidemiological research would be impossible. We would have no way of finding out whether mental illness was commoner in one culture than another, or whether its incidence and manifestations varied with other factors like poverty, social class and ethnic background. Without a criterion for distinguishing between sickness and health, and between one sort of sickness and another, there could never be any rational planning of psychiatric services. Indeed all scientific communication would be impossible and our professional journals would be restricted to individual case reports, anecdotes and statements of opinion.

The clinician, who deals with one patient at a time, may succeed in convincing himself that he does not and need not classify his patients, but even here, as we have seen, this is not really so unless he is offering the same treatment to everyone he sees. The research worker and administrator, who deal with populations of patients rather than individuals, cannot even pretend to avoid classification. There is no point in defining a population unless its members possess something in common with one another which distinguish them from members of other populations, and once this condition has been satisfied a classification has been created.

I would like to emphasize, though, that this argument, which I believe to be irrefutable, is in no sense a denial of the value of the comprehensive formulation of the individual patient's predicament which Menninger and others have advocated, nor is it a brusque dismissal of their criticisms of the shortcomings of our existing classifications and of the ways in which we use them. It is undeniable that a diagnosis *by itself* is almost never an adequate basis for treating an individual patient. It will probably set limits to what it is possible, or necessary, to achieve, and exclude some forms of treatment from consideration, but a host of other factors, the patient's personality, his relationships with other people, his reasons for seeking treatment, his social background and so on, will all influence one's aims and the ways in which one seeks to achieve them. The complexity of the situation can only be dealt with adequately by a comprehensive analysis.

SHORTCOMINGS AND HARMFUL EFFECTS IN PERSPECTIVE

However, not all the criticisms that have been levelled at psychiatric diagnoses are valid, and others have been overstated. It is true that a diagnosis may provide little definite information about the patient's prognosis' or even about his symptoms or how he should be treated, but at the very least it has the important negative function of excluding from consideration many other types of problem. To know that a patient has a depressive neurosis at least tells us that he is not elated, or deluded, or hallucinated; that the question of compulsory detention in hospital does not arise; and that he is sad and unhappy for reasons that seem understandable. It is undeniable that psychiatric diagnoses are often unreliable, and that it is commonplace for a single patient to be given three different diagnoses by three different psychiatrists, but this does not have to be so. It has been demonstrated several times that adequately trained psychiatrists can achieve acceptable levels of agreement, and that there are consistent differences in symptomatology, course and response to treatment between populations of patients from different diagnostic categories. It has to be admitted that the names we give our illnesses sometimes encourage facile assumptions about disease entities and causes, what Cohen (1953) called a 'penny in the slot machine' approach to diagnosis, but this problem also can be dealt with by educating doctors without abandoning diagnosis. As to the belief that attributing a diagnosis to a patient somehow detracts from his dignity as a human being, it is surely the role that matters rather than the diagnosis. It is being a patient, and particularly a psychiatric patient, that hurts, rather than being regarded as a manic depressive. Without changing society's attitudes to mental illness and other forms of deviance it is difficult to see how abandoning diagnoses would help very much. Although it is true that several of our diagnostic terms, like hysteric and psychopath, have acquired pejorative connotations even amongst psychiatrists, these connotations exist because they denote ways of being mentally ill, or failing to cope. It is the fact that the patient is crazy, or manipulative, or unable to cope with the demands of everyday life, that creates the odium, not the diagnosis itself. And, although the use of diagnostic labels may indeed make it easier for psychiatrists to lose sight of the fact that their patients are also people with ordinary human feelings, they also enable them to recognize them as schizophrenics or manic depressives and give them the appropriate treatment. Acceptance and understanding are valuable, but so too is recognition and if there has to be a choice between the two, the latter may well be more important in the main areas of psychiatric practice.

CONCLUSIONS

In summary then, psychiatric diagnoses have serious shortcomings. They sometimes bring other disadvantages in their train and they are liable to be misused in various ways. But none of these is an intrinsic defect of all classifications, nor is any tool safe from the risk of misuse. As with any other innovation, the advantages and disadvantages of a classification of psychiatric disorders have to be balanced against one another. The advantage of a classification is quite simply that it allows us to communicate.

The following chapters take these conclusions as their starting point. From this point on it will be taken as proven that psychiatry cannot function at all without classifying its subject matter. It will also be regarded as self-evident that our present classifications are imperfect, and also misused. What follows is essentially a description of our existing Kraepelinean classification, with its strengths and weaknesses, its uses and failings, followed by a discussion of some of the ways in which it could be improved, and an outline of some of the alternative forms of classification with which it might be replaced.

# 2 The Nature of Disease and Diagnosis

## DEFINITIONS OF DISEASE

There is no concept in medicine more fundamental than that of disease or illness. Everyone, physician and layman alike, uses the words and takes it for granted that their meaning is self-evident and unambiguous. Perhaps because they are so commonplace little thought is ever given to them and they are rarely defined except in dictionaries. Occasionally, arguments develop about whether or not a particular phenomenon, like alcoholism or homosexuality, is a disease, but even these rarely lead to a search for a definition. Laymen tend to feel uneasily that only physicians can be expected to answer such questions; and physicians are either so convinced that the answer is yes, or alternatively no, that no thought is necessary, or else plead that no answer is possible in our present state of knowledge. Rarely does anyone suggest, particularly to a medical audience, that the answer depends on what is meant by disease. In fact, as Scadding (1963) has pointed out, all sorts of problems result from our failure to define fundamental terms clearly enough, and the worst confusion is always caused by terms that are so familiar that we are hardly aware that any assumptions are involved in using them.

Even when allowance is made for the essentially empirical nature of medicine, and the impatience with theorizing and philosophizing that such an atmosphere engenders, it is remarkable how little thought has been given to deciding exactly what 'disease' is, and what properties diseases should and should not possess. Most physicians rarely give such matters a moment's thought, even though they may well unwittingly use the words disease and illness in different senses at different times, or get involved in disputes produced by unrecognized differences in the meaning attributed to them. Psychiatrists are usually more aware than others of some of the problems involved, because the forensic decision to remove the burden of criminal responsibility from the mentally ill frequently involves them in having to decide whether people are ill or not, and to justify their decisions to hard-headed lawyers; but they have not been conspicuously successful in finding solutions. It is important to appreciate, though, that these problems do not apply only to psychiatry. The whole of medicine is in much the same predicament, or would be if important legal decisions hinged on the issue.

It is not so much a definition we lack as an adequate one. Numerous definitions of disease have been suggested from time to time, but the majority are either hopelessly vague, or tautologous, or exclude people who, by common consent, are ill or include others who, by the same token, are not. Most of the definitions offered in dictionaries, including medical ones, define disease either as a state of sickness or impaired health, which hardly advances the matter very far, or in terms of a disturbance of function, leaving it unclear how the presence of a disturbance is to be recognized. The definition in the current (24th) edition of Dorland's *Illustrated Medical Dictionary* ('A definite morbid process having a characteristic train of symptoms . . .') is representative of the former, and that in the *Shorter Oxford English Dictionary* ('a condition of the body, or of some part or organ of the body, in which its functions are disturbed or deranged') of the latter.

DISEASE AS SUFFERING

Historically there can be little doubt that the concept of disease originated as an explanation for the onset of suffering and incapacity in the absence of obvious injury, that the concept of health was a later development, implying the absence of disease. Naturally enough, therefore, attempts have often been made to define illness in terms of suffering or incapacity, or at least in terms of a complaint of some sort. However, this immediately leads to difficulties. Many people who are ill, even physically ill, do not complain or suffer, either because they experience no symptoms, or because they ignore what in others would be cause for complaint, or simply because they drop dead without warning. A man with a cancer growing silently in his lung, or someone with cardiac pain which he dismisses as 'a touch of wind' would both be regarded by doctors and laymen as ill, and urgently in need of treatment, yet neither complains, or even suffers to any significant extent. The same is true of the manic patient who has never felt better in his life, or the schizophrenic who is unshakably convinced that his voices are real, or the typhoid carrier harbouring salmonellae in his gall bladder. Other people complain incessantly, and insist that they suffer, without either their doctors or anyone else being convinced that they are genuinely ill.

DISEASE IS WHAT DOCTORS TREAT

Partly because of problems of this sort Kraupl Taylor (1971) has suggested that what he calls 'therapeutic concern' would be a more appropriate criterion; people would be regarded as ill, in other words, if either they or others were convinced they needed medical attention. A criterion of this sort would certainly be capable of embracing people whom doctors, or society as a whole, regarded as in need of treatment as well as those who complained or suffered personally, but in doing so it would create a worse problem than the one it solved. Equating llness with a complaint allows the individual to be sole arbiter of whether he is ill or not. This is unsatisfactory because some people who should be complaining don't do so, and others who do so repeatedly don't seem to have adequate reasons for doing so. Equating illness with other people's 'therapeutic concern' implies that no one can be ill until he has been recognized as such, and also gives doctors, and society, free rein to label all deviants as ill, thus opening the door to all the inconsistencies and abuses Szasz has vividly conjured up.

The fact is that any definition of disease that boils down to 'what people complain of' or 'what doctors treat', or some combination of the two, is almost worse than no definition at all. It is free to expand or contract with changes in social attitudes and therapeutic optimism and is at the mercy of idiosyncratic judgements by doctors or patients. If one wished to compare the incidence of disease in two different cultures, or in a single population at two different times, whose criteria of suffering or therapeutic concern would one use? And if the results of a study comparing the amount of sickness in a society at two different times suggested that the incidence of illness had risen, would this be because people's health had deteriorated, or because their attitudes to illness had changed?

## DISEASE AS A LESION

The development first of morbid anatomy and then of histology in the 19th century produced widespread evidence that illness was often accompanied by structural damage to the body, either at a gross or a microscopic level. It was only a short step from this observation to the assumption that these lesions constituted the illness, and that illness necessarily involved structural damage. Subsequently, as knowledge of biochemistry and physiology caught up with that of anatomy, this concept was expanded to include evidence of a biochemical or physiological abnormality, without relinquishing the basic assumption that illness necessarily involved a demonstrable physical abnormality of some sort.

In this 19th century milieu it was almost inevitable that the presence of an identifiable lesion should come to be regarded as the hallmark or defining characteristic of disease, and this concept of illness was, explicitly or implicitly, dominant until quite recently. Such a standpoint does indeed have many advantages. It provides an objective criterion which is not at the mercy of changing social attitudes and therapeutic fashions, and also embodies at least a partial explanation of the patient's symptoms or disabilities. On close examination, however, a number of problems arise. The concept of an abnormality or a lesion is quite straightforward so long as one is concerned with a departure from a standard pattern. But as soon as we begin to recognize that there is no single standard pattern of structure or function, and that even healthy human beings and all their constituent tissues and organs vary considerably in size, shape, composition and functional efficiency, it becomes much less obvious what constitutes a lesion, where normal variation ends and abnormality begins. Is, for instance, hypertension a disease, and if so what is the level beyond which the blood pressure is 'abnormal'? Is shortsightedness to be regarded as a disease? And what of minor congenital abnormalities, like fused second and third toes and albinism? An even more serious problem is that symptoms whose physical basis has not yet been demonstrated cannot be accepted as diseases. Trigeminal neuralgia, senile pruritus, proctalgia fugax, dystonia musculorum, even migraine, must all be discarded. Fifty years ago, the same would have been true of most forms of epilepsy, Parkinson's disease, chorea, Bornholm disease and most deliria.

Insistence on the presence of a demonstrable lesion causes particular problems for psychiatry as no physical basis has yet been identified for most of its major syndromes. For this reason, the majority of psychiatrists have baulked at accepting any such criterion, though a few have done so with enthusiasm. Kurt Schneider (1950) willingly accepted that the word illness should only be used in situations in which 'some actual morbid change' or 'defective structure' was present in the body, and stated bluntly that he did not regard either neurotic states or personality disorders as illness, but simply as 'abnormal varieties of sane mental life'. However, he still regarded schizophrenia and manic depressive psychosis as illness, along with organic and toxic psychoses, on the basis of a convenient but unjustifiable assumption that in time they would prove to have an 'underlying morbid physical condition'. Szasz (1960) has gone further, taking Schneider's argument to its logical conclusion and maintaining that, as they lack any demonstrable physical basis, there cannot be any such thing as mental illnesses and that to speak of illness in this context is to use the word in a purely metaphorical sense.

DISEASE AS ADAPTATION TO STRESS

For understandable reasons, the reaction against the 19th century's 'physical lesion' concept of illness was led by psychiatrists, particularly by Adolph Meyer in Baltimore. Meyer insisted that diseases, especially mental ones, were reactions of the whole organism to its total environment, rather than noxae attacking it from without or structural lesions within. He was also at pains to emphasize that, as every individual is unique, and his environment likewise, the reaction which constituted his disease must also be unique. The theme was taken up enthusiastically by his numerous pupils. Seguin (1946) proposed that disease should be formally defined as 'a reaction of the organism as a whole to external or internal stimuli altering seriously its equilibrium' and reiterated that a patient's disease 'can only be considered as a unique phenomenon, and handled as such'.

A definition of this sort, emphasizing the differences between one sick individual and another rather than their similarities, obviously hampers attempts to classify diseases, but an even more serious problem is that it fails to provide any criterion for distinguishing between sickness and health, or disease and non-disease. It would be quite reasonable to define life itself as a series of reactions by the organism to external or internal stimuli. How then is one to distinguish between those which 'alter seriously its equilibrium' and those which do not? Seguin's own criterion that equilibrium is seriously altered 'when the organism cannot recover from it' is clearly inadequate, as it would appear to exclude all illnesses normally ending in full recovery. Alternatively, if it does not do this, it provides no means of distinguishing between temporary disturbances which are to be regarded as disease and those, like the breathlessness, tachycardia and metabolic acidosis produced by exercise, which are not.

## DISEASE AS IMPERFECTION

Health and sickness, like good and evil, and light and dark, constitute a single bipolar concept in the sense that they are the antithesis of one another. The presence of either excludes the other or, more precisely, any increase in the one diminishes the other.

This means that whenever we determine the extent or degree to which someone is sick, in doing so, we automatically determine how healthy he is as well. It also means that concepts or definitions of sickness carry with them implicit concepts or definitions of health, and vice versa. If sickness is defined by the presence of a 'lesion', any human condition in which no lesion is to be found is by definition healthy. And if all departures from normality, all imperfections, are regarded as forms of illness, then the only truly healthy state is one of perfection. The most influential conceptual system of this latter kind is psychoanalytic theory. According to this theory, the unavoidable vicissitudes of early life activate morbid psychological mechanisms which impair personality development and functioning in everyone to a greater or lesser extent. Although these handicaps are regarded as potentially reversible if appropriate treatment is provided, this implicitly reduces health to an idealized state of complete normality, an almost hypothetical state to which man can only aspire, and some degree of sickness becomes his universal lot. There is, to be sure, nothing inherently absurd or illogical in this, but it does carry profound implications for society's attitudes towards the sick, for individuals' attitudes to themselves, and not least for the staffing and financing of medical services. On all these counts a more restricted concept of sickness seems preferable. The definition of health as 'a state of complete physical, mental and social wellbeing' enshrined in the charter of the World Health Organization has similar implications, although in view of its setting, it is probably wiser to regard this particular statement as a fine ringing phrase intended to epitomize the political aspirations of a great international organization rather than as a practical definition.

A STATISTICAL CONCEPT OF DISEASE

Although psychiatrists were the first to protest about the short-comings of the 19th century's lesion/pathogen concept of disease, these eventually became apparent to others also. When Pickering and his colleagues (Oldham, Pickering, Fraser Roberts and Sowry, 1960) demonstrated beyond reasonable doubt that such a major cause of death and disability as essential hypertension was a graded characteristic, dependent like height and intelligence on polygenic inheritance and shading insensibly into normality, it was clear that a new concept of illness was required, and that this would have to be based on a statistical model of the relationship between normality and abnormality. In fact, Cohen (1943) had foreseen this some years before by defining disease simply as 'deviation from the normal . . . . by way of excess or defect'. Indeed, Broussais and Magendie had come close to doing the same thing a hundred years earlier. But in spite of its statistical basis – from the general tenor of his essay – one must assume that he was using the term normal in a statistical rather than in an ideal sense – Cohen's definition is still inadequate. This is mainly because, as it stands, it does not distinguish between deviations from the norm which are harmful, like hypertension, those which are neutral, like great height, and those which are positively beneficial, like superior intelligence. Scadding (1967) has attempted to deal with this problem by stipulating that the abnormal phenomena must place the affected individual at a 'biological disadvantage', reducing either his chances of survival or his chances of procreation. As the formal definition of disease he offers is based on a very careful consideration of the many problems and issues involved, and is certainly less unsatisfactory than any of the alternatives mentioned previously, it is worth studying in detail.

SCADDING'S DEFINITION

Scadding defines a disease as 'the sum of the abnormal phenomena displayed by a group of living organisms in association with a specified common characteristic or set of characteristics by which they differ from the norm for their species in such a way as to place them at a biological disadvantage'.

Although this is a definition of *a* disease, rather than of the global concept of disease, it has a number of fundamental implications for the latter. The most important of these is that it is based on Cohen's idea of deviation from the norm of the species, set out in more explicitly statistical terms. This statistical basis is the crux of the matter, for it carries with it several fundamental implications – that deviation in either direction, too much or too little, is equally capable of producing disease; that the boundary between sickness and health may need to be an arbitrary one, like the boundary between mental subnormality and normal intelligence; and that the majority are automatically debarred from being regarded as ill. The 'specified common characteristic or set of characteristics' is the defining characteristic of the individual disease in question. Its presence is essential for establishing the presence of that disease, and it is worth noting in passing that Scadding's wording allows it to be either monothetic (a single trait) or polythetic (a set of traits, no one of which is mandatory). The concept of biological disadvantage is obviously a useful one, though it is less unambiguous than it seems. Although any increase in mortality or reduction in fertility are presumably adequate to establish its presence, it is unclear whether disabilities which are either too slight to affect mortality or too late developing to impair fertility can also qualify. Moreover, what is a disadvantage to the individual may not always be so to the population to which he belongs, and it is not clear whose disadvantage, the individual's or the group's, should take precedence. Problems of this sort are particularly important where social animals like man are concerned. Homosexuality, for instance, is undoubtedly a biological disadvantage to the individual by virtue of drastically reducing his chances of procreating. But if it could be shown that homosexuals possessed valuable aptitudes which others lacked, it could be argued quite plausibly that a community which contained a proportion of homosexuals might have competitive advantages over those that did not. Indeed, in an era of explosive population growth like that which our species is currently experiencing, it may be biologically advantageous to a community to have its fertility reduced anyway.

This is simply one example of a more general problem. A characteristic which is a disadvantage in one environment may be beneficial in another. The sickle cell trait is a deviation from the norm which in most environments produces a slight but definite biological disadvantage. In an environment in which malaria is endemic, however, it is positively beneficial. Is it then to be regarded as an illness in the first environment but not in the second? Such problems as this arise because the environment, with its capacity to tilt the scales one way or the other, is ignored in Scadding's definition. This is a particularly serious matter where mental illness is concerned because here the environment, and especially its social aspects, is often of paramount importance. Qualities like recklessness and aggressiveness, for example, may lead a man to be regarded as a psychopath in one environment and to be admired as a hero in another. Of course, it could be argued very reasonably that social advantages or disadvantages of this kind are irrelevant, and that the disadvantage is specified as being a biological one for this reason. But it is not always easy to decide where a biological disadvantage ends and a social one begins, or to visualize a human environment shorn of all social components.

The key phrase in Scadding's definition, 'the sum of the abnormal phenomena', may also be difficult to apply where mental illness is concerned. For most physical illnesses, the norm is fairly clearly established because the relevant physiological mechanisms are reasonably well understood. We know a great deal about the normal functioning of the heart and kidney and so find it relatively easy to decide what is abnormal and what is not. We know much less about normal psychological functioning and find it correspondingly harder to distinguish between the normal and the pathological. It is more difficult than we like to admit, for instance, to distinguish between normal grief and a pathological reaction to bereavement, or between a delusion and an overvalued idea. Where an abnormality of part function is involved, as in these two examples, the situation is not too desperate. We have psychological criteria of a sort available for assessing normality. However, where the only abnormal phenomena involve the total behaviour of the individual, and the abnormality is essentially a departure from a social or moral norm, we are soon adrift. As Lewis (1953) has emphasized, once we allow social norms to become our criterion of normality all socially deviant or disapproved behaviour becomes liable to be regarded as sickness. Lewis's own solution to this quandary was to insist that our criterion of abnormality where mental illness was concerned should be firmly rooted in a disturbance of psychological functioning, in the same way that our criterion of physical abnormality is rooted in a disturbance of physiological function. The snag is that at present we know so little psychology that this course can be little more than an aspiration. In many areas, if we are determined not to resort to social criteria, all we can do is defer judgement.

Many of these problems are obviously caused by the short-comings of psychology and psychiatry, rather than by those of Scadding's definition. But they do illustrate the difficulties of applying even so carefully thought out a definition as this within the realm of mental illness. Certainly, they provide little grounds for confidence in expecting formal definitions of disease to provide us with a firm criterion for deciding whether the psychopath and the exhibitionist are ill or not, or for distinguishing the phobias, mood changes and rituals of neurotic illness from the fears, fancies and idiosyncracies of normal health.

DISEASE AS A PLAN OF ACTION

An alternative way of elucidating the meaning of the word disease, or illness, is to examine how it is used in practice. If one does this, it soon becomes apparent that there are many situations in which everyone is agreed that a disease is present, and others where the question of illness does not arise at all. But there are also a number of areas in which physicians disagree amongst themselves. Where mental illness is concerned, the main disputed area is the general field of personality disorder, together with the related phenomena of sexual deviation, alcoholism and drug abuse. Physical disorders generally give rise to less disagreement, but a symptom-free typhoid carrier, a woman with a carcinoma-in-situ of the cervix, a child with a congenital club foot, or anyone complaining of pain for which no cause can be found, are all liable to be regarded as ill by some doctors but not by others. In such cases, it will almost invariably be found that those who regard the subject as ill also regard some medical procedure, treatment or investigation, as necessary, while those who do not regard the subject as ill do not regard either treatment or investigation as warranted. This gives rise to the suspicion that the answer one gets to the question 'Is this a disease?' is really a covert answer to the quite different question 'Should this person be under medical care?' As Linder has put it, a diagnosis is not a description, an explanation, or even a prediction, it is simply a disguised prescription (Linder, 1965).

Linder has also drawn attention to one significant exception to this principle which is of particular importance to psychiatry. In any situation in which a man's behaviour infringes the law, or is offensive to others in more general ways, he is normally liable to be blamed, or even punished, but if he is deemed to be mentally ill this is no longer so. Explicitly in the case of the criminal law, and in practice also in the case of public attitudes, mental illness excuses behaviour which would otherwise invite blame and retribution. In any setting in which this issue arises, in a court of law or not, physicians may disagree about whether the subject is ill because they disagree about whether it is appropriate for him to be held responsible for his behaviour. In other words, there are some settings in which the statement that an individual is or is not ill may be a covert answer to the question 'Should he be held responsible for his behaviour?' rather than to the usual question 'Should he be under medical care?'.

Although this formulation takes no account of the routine involvement of physicians in essentially physiological processes like childbirth, and more recent incursions into other areas like family planning, it is difficult to refute Linder's basic argument. Indeed, in some ways it clarifies the problem by implying that disagreements about what is or is not illness are not really logical or semantic disagreements at all, but simply empirical disagreements over the issue of whether, in a given case, medical procedures are likely to be beneficial. Among other things, it explains why such disagreements are commoner in psychiatry than in other branches of medicine. They are more common simply because there is more uncertainty about the efficacy of the therapeutic measures employed in psychiatry than there is elsewhere. If, for example, the effectiveness of the various techniques used in the treatment of personality disorders was established one way or the other, we would probably no longer disagree about whether personality disorders were illnesses or not.

This view of diagnosis as a disguised plan of action obviously has much in common with the 'disease is what doctors treat' argument, or Kraupl Taylor's criterion of 'therapeutic concern', but there is a crucial difference. Kraupl Taylor is advocating the presence or absence of 'therapeutic concern' as a workable criterion for the presence or absence of illness or, as he would call it, 'patienthood'. Linder is arguing that we have no consistent criterion for the presence of illness, but disguise the fact by substituting the purely practical issue of whether or not medical attention is appropriate.

### Scadding's definition or Linder's argument?

Assuming that this is an accurate analysis of the situation, we are faced with a choice between adopting Scadding's definition of disease, or some modification of it, and trying to develop a set of working rules from this statement of principles, or alternatively accepting Linder's argument that we do not possess any concept of illness other than the purely empirical concept of what, in any given state of therapeutic optimism and ability, is a fit subject for medical attention. Which of the two we accept will almost inevitably be determined by the context. In any situation in which we need to measure the amount of illness in a population, either to compare one population with another or to measure change within a single population over time, we must have a definition of disease which is independent of therapeutic innovations and fashions. This means that we must use Scadding's definition, or something comparable, or abandon our task. But in the everyday situation where we are concerned with the subject matter of medicine, rather than with disease, we can afford to accept Linder's argument. This is so because in practice, it is not necessary to decide precisely what illness is in order to classify illnesses. This is well illustrated by the fact that none of the three glossaries to the current (8th) edition of the Mental Disorders section of the *International Classification*, American, British or WHO, makes any attempts to define 'mental disorder' in spite of the fact that they are all concerned with the classification of its various manifestations. Nor do they even remark on their failure to do so, though the British glossary does comment on its failure to define the term 'psychosis', adding significantly that 'no such definition is required for the effective use of the classification' (General Register Office, 1968). This singular omission might well strike taxonomists as surprising, even shocking, and certainly the lack of a definition allows the territory embraced by the terms mental illness and mental disorder to expand or contract in unpredictable ways. But it can legitimately be argued that, in practice, medical classifications need this freedom because they need to embrace all those whom physicians encounter in the patient role, regardless of whether they are ill or not. If otherwise healthy people whose marriages are threatening to break up frequently seek help from psychiatrists, then psychiatric classifications need to be constructed to accommodate such people, and the same applies to adolescents referred to psychiatrists by courts because they are taking drugs, or children brought by their parents for starting fires. The corollary to this, which is not as widely recognized as it should be, is that it does not necessarily follow because someone has been examined by a psychiatrist, allocated to a diagnostic category and offered treatment, that they are or ever were mentally ill.

DEFINITIONS OF INDIVIDUAL DISEASES

If we have no adequate definition of disease as a global concept, it becomes even more important to have adequate definitions for individual diseases. Unfortunately, as soon as one begins to consider individual illnesses, it becomes apparent that there is no consistent theme. Some, like tuberculosis, are defined by their cause, others, like ulcerative colitis, by their pathology, others, like migraine, by their symptoms, and so on. The reasons for this state of affairs lie in the historical development of the global concept of disease we have just been considering. To the Cnidean School of the ancient world symptoms and signs were themselves diseases. Fever, asthma, joint pains and skin rashes were all separate diseases to be studied individually, and this assumption persisted until very recently. Most of the 2400 diseases Boissier de Sauvages described in the 18th century were merely individual symptoms. The idea of disease as a syndrome, a constellation of related symptoms with a characteristic prognosis – to remit, to evolve or to persist – originated with Sydenham in the 17th century, though the Greek Empiricist school had had the germ of the idea long before. This concept lasted until the early 19th century when Morgagni and Bichat popularized post mortem dissection of the body as a routine procedure, and so converted disease from a clinical entity observed at the bedside to a characteristic morbid anatomy observed in the cadaver. Thereafter, new concepts followed one another in rapid progression mainly, as Feinstein (1969) has pointed out, in response to the introduction of new types of observational technology. With the development of powerful microscopes in the middle of the 19th century, individual cells could be examined as well as tissues and whole organs, and the consequent detection of cellular pathology led Virchow and his contemporaries to assume that cellular derangements were the basis of all disease. This concept was, in its turn, displaced by the discovery of bacteria by Koch and Pasteur, a development that was responsible more than anything else for the concept of 'disease entities' each produced by a single aetiological agent. Currently, new techniques like electrophoresis, chromosomal analysis and electron microscopy are producing yet further concepts of disease expressed in terms of deranged biophysical structures, genes and molecules. As Riese (1953) aptly observed, the history of medicine could be written in terms of man's changing concept of disease.

Each of these waves of technology has added new diseases and from each stage some have survived, so the diseases which figure in contemporary textbooks have a very variable conceptual basis. A few, like senile pruritus and proctalgia fugax, are simply Cnidean symptoms, even though first described relatively recently. Others, like migraine and most of the diseases of psychiatry, are clinical syndromes, Sydenham's constellation of symptoms. Mitral stenosis and cholelithiasis are based on morbid anatomy, and tumours of all kinds on histopathology.

Tuberculosis and syphilis are based on bacteriology and the concept of the aetiological agent, prophyria on biochemistry, myasthenia gravis on physiological dysfunction, Down's syndrome on chromosomal architecture, and so on. In fact, our present classification is rather like an old mansion which has been refurnished many times, but always without clearing out the old furniture first, so that amongst the new inflatable plastic settees and glass coffee tables are still scattered a few old Tudor stools, Jacobean dressers and Regency commodes, and a great deal of Victoriana. Indeed, Scadding is probably close to the truth when he suggests that it is this logical heterogeniety in our definitions of individual diseases that is responsible for our inability to produce a satisfactory definition of disease as a whole (Scadding, 1972).

An even older and more influential relic from the past is the assumption that diseases are intangible noxae, which silently and mysteriously attack the individual from without. All cultures recognize at least some forms of incapacity and suffering as disease and most, including our own until recently, attribute these to malign supernatural influences. Whether it be a witches' spell, divine retribution, or the invisible effluvia of swamps and marshes, in all three the theme is essentially the same. Something mysterious, intangible and alien is responsible. The discovery of bacteria in the latter half of the 19th century suddenly endowed this deeply rooted cultural belief with scientific respectability. Seguin (1946) has referred to the bacterial era as 'the Golden Age for the demoniac concept of disease' and there is no doubt that the combination of these two, the half dormant cultural tradition and the power and prestige of science, served to reinforce and perpetuate the implicit assumption that all diseases were entities of some sort, attacking the individual from without and possessing some kind of shadowy independent existence of their own.

The diversity of conceptual basis to which I have referred is accompanied by a matching diversity of defining characteristics. The concept of a disease cholelithiasis arose at a time when diseases were regarded as disturbances of normal anatomy and so its defining characteristic was, and still remains, anatomical, namely the presence of stones in the gall bladder. Similarly, the concept of tuberculosis (as opposed to the much more limited concept of phthisis) developed in an era when infection by a specific micro-organism was the paradigm of disease so its defining characteristic was, and still is, the presence of the tubercle bacillus, regardless of what the patient's symptoms are or what part of his body is affected. Sometimes, however, the defining characteristic of an illness changes as knowledge of its antecedents increases, and this change may be accompanied by a subtle and sometimes unrecognized change in the population of patients to whom the diagnosis applies. Scadding (1963) quotes the example of myxodema which was originally defined by its syndrome, but came to be defined by a disorder of function, a deficiency in the production or utilization of thyroxine. This new defining characteristic includes some patients, those with hypopituitarism, who were not embraced by the original criterion, and excludes others, those with localized myxoedema in the absence of hypothyroidism, who were. Changes of this sort are not a problem provided they are explicit, but often they take place slowly over many years and during the transition period it is often unclear which disease is being referred to, the old or the new. A further complication resulting from diseases being defined on several different levels is that individual patients may meet the defining characteristics of two or three different diseases simultaneously, their symptomatology qualifying them for one disease, a disorder of function for a second, and an anatomical lesion for a third. A man with a bad chest, for instance, may qualify for a diagnosis of chronic bronchitis by virtue of having a chronic productive cough, for a diagnosis of asthma by being intermittently breathless as a result of variable bronchiolar narrowing, and for a diagnosis of emphysema because his pulmonary alveoli are dilated.

Such problems as these, resulting from the variable and changeable basis of the defining characteristics of different diseases, are less serious where mental illness is concerned than in most other branches of medicine because the majority of psychiatric illnesses, and all the so-called functional illnesses, are defined at the same clinical–descriptive level. The dominant conceptual model of illness in psychiatry is still the syndrome model Sydenham introduced in the 17th century, a cluster of symptoms and signs with a characteristic time course. Although in many ways this is lamentable, a cause of low reliability and witness to our ignorance, the fact that most diagnoses are defined on the same basis does at least enable psychiatry to avoid problems of this particular kind.

DISEASES AS CONCEPTS

Several times in this discussion diseases have been referred to as concepts, and reference has been made to the way in which a change in the defining characteristics of a disease may alter the population of patients embraced by the term, and even their symptoms and signs. One might add too, that it is commonplace for old concepts like Banti's syndrome and shell shock to die out, just as it is for new ones like primary aldosteronism and trisomy 21 to come into existence. In view of all this, it is well nigh impossible for us to regard illnesses as having any sort of independent material existence. To our generation it is self-evident that diseases, tuberculosis as well as schizophrenia, are nothing but man made abstractions, inventions justified only by their convenience and liable at any time to be adjusted or discarded. Our present outlook is so wholeheartedly empirical that we find it difficult to credit how an earlier generation could have talked of diseases being 'discovered' like so many golden sovereigns on a beach, or have imagined that there were a finite number of them waiting to be identified. Yet although we know these things perfectly well, we have still not rid ourselves of all the old Platonic assumptions. Claims are still made even now that this or that syndrome is a 'disease entity', in spite of the fact that the word entity, defined in the Oxford dictionary as a 'thing that has real existence', is meaningless outside its original Platonic context. Similarly, the suggestion that patients with, for example, both schizophrenic and affective symptoms ought perhaps to be regarded as genuine interforms half way between schizophrenia and manic depressive illness still meets with expressions of shock or incredulity, as if they must really have one or other illness even if their symptoms are atypical. Part of the problem lies in the tendency of all concepts to become 'reified' and for familiarity to lead to their origins in human imagination being forgotten. The concepts of physics are as prone to this tendency as those of medicine and it may be that we are up against some of the inherent limitations of our conceptual abilities.

THE 'NON-EXISTENCE' ARGUMENT

Just at present, however, we are probably in greater danger of discarding our disease concepts completely than we are of attributing material existence to them. The pendulum has swung so far that concepts like schizophrenia and psychopathy are now in greater danger of dismissal than of reification. Szasz, Laing and others have repeatedly and gleefully asserted that 'there is no such thing as schizophrenia' or that 'schizophrenia does not exist' and been loudly applauded, at least in non-medical circles, for doing so. It is, of course, perfectly true that schizophrenia is a concept rather than an object of our senses. But the same is equally true of all other concepts, including tuberculosis and migraine, and good and evil. The fact that tuberculosis does not exist in a material sense does not prevent men dying because their lungs have been destroyed by the tubercle bacillus, nor does it relieve his headache to tell a man that there is no such thing as migraine. So it is with schizophrenia also. Even if Eugen Bleuler had never coined the term, the behavioural abnormalities, the personal experiences and the biological disadvantages which we associate with it would have remained unchanged. It is true, as Scheff (1963) and other sociologists have pointed out, that part of the disability and suffering accompanying conditions like schizophrenia is a result of the individual being labelled and treated as a schizophrenic by other people, but it is simply mischievous to suggest that schizophrenia is nothing more than the product of social or intrafamilial pressures of this kind. In fact it is equally meaningless to assert on behalf of any abstract noun or concept either that it does or that it does not exist. The only question at issue is whether it is a useful concept, and even this question has to be asked within a defined context. For the forseeable future, the usefulness of the concept of schizophrenia is amply established by the universal occurrence of the behavioural and experiential anomalies to which the term refers, irrespective of differences in language and culture; by the biological disadvantage associated with these anomalies, again irrespective of language or culture; by the evidence that these abnormalities are, at least in part, transmitted genetically; and by the influence on them of drugs which lack analogous effects on other people. It may well be that in time the term will lose its usefulness and pass out of use, as earlier concepts like dropsy and monomania have done, but if it does so it will be because it has been replaced by other more useful concepts, not because of any sudden realization that there is no such thing.

## DIAGNOSIS

From time to time in this discussion of the concept of disease, reference has been made to the act of diagnosis and sometimes diseases have been referred to as diagnoses. The word diagnosis is derived from the Greek words διά (two) and γιγνώσκειν (to know or perceive) and means literally to distinguish or to differentiate. In the medical context with which we are concerned it is used both as a verb and as a noun. The former describes the decision process by which a particular disease is attributed to a particular patient, in preference to any of the other diseases potentially applicable to him, and the latter is the decision reached, the actual illness attributed to that individual.

### THE LOGIC OF CLASS MEMBERSHIP

At first sight this appears to be a straightforward exercise in determining class membership in accordance with the traditional rules of logic. In fact this is far from being the case, but it may still be helpful to describe these rules and the assumptions they involve, if only to illustrate some of the problems which diagnosis involves. The ideal abstract classes of the logician are mutually exclusive and jointly exhaustive; that is, every member of the universe possesses the defining attributes of one class of the set or array and none possesses the defining attributes of more than one. The defining attributes of the classes, and the attributes of all their members, are also 'exact', meaning that they are either present or absent, and never present in partial form. Determining the attributes of the individual and knowing the defining attributes of all the classes in the set are therefore all that is necessary to allocate the individual to the appropriate class. One might visualize, for instance, a classification of geometrical figures. Each class in the set, triangles, parallelograms, trapezoids, and so on, would be defined by the number of its sides and the angles between them. Every figure in the universe under consideration would possess the attributes of one of these classes, i.e. figures whose sides were curved or bent would automatically be excluded. Thus, counting the number of sides possessed by an individual figure and measuring the angles between these would be sufficient to determine its class membership, regardless of how many sides it possessed.

EMPIRICAL CLASSES

All real or empirical classes depart from this abstract ideal in some respects. First, they are often 'polythetic' rather than 'monothetic', meaning that they are defined not by a single necessary attribute, but by the presence of some or most of a number of attributes, none of which is mandatory for class membership. The Mammalia, for instance, are characterized by the fact that they are warm blooded, deliver their young alive, suckle them with specialized mammary glands, and possess hair and a single mandible that articulates directly with the skull. The fact that an animal lacks one or two of these characteristics does not necessarily mean that it is not a mammal, provided it possesses the others. Secondly, empirical classes are often 'inexact', meaning that their defining characteristics are capable of quantitative variation, rather than only being present or absent, so that as a result members of the domain cannot always be allocated with confidence to membership or non-membership. To pursue the same example as before, the platypus is neither cold blooded like the reptiles nor genuinely warm blooded like other mammals, but half way between the two. It maintains its body temperature above that of its environment, but is unable to keep it constant in the face of environmental fluctuations.

CLASSIFICATION OF DISEASES

Diseases share both these shortcomings of empirical classes in general. They also raise novel problems of their own. In other biological classifications it can generally be assumed quite safely that every individual belongs to one class in the array and cannot belong to two classes simultaneously, or belong to one class at one time and to another later on. The six-legged creature crawling across your desk will always belong to some insect species or other. It will not be both a beetle and a butterfly, or a beetle at one stage in its life and a butterfly at another. None of these assumptions is justified where diseases are concerned. The reason for this is that making a diagnosis is not simply a matter of allocating a human being to the appropriate class, as would be the case if he were being allocated to a species or ethnic group. Nor is it a matter of allocating an individual disease to the appropriate generic category, because a disease can only exist in the context of a diseased person. In other words, when we make a diagnosis we are not classifying people, or diseases, but sick people, and any individual person may be diseased in different ways either at different times or simultaneously. Thus, in any given instance in which the question of making a diagnosis arises, there will generally be several possibilities. It may be appropriate to make one diagnosis (e.g. chronic bronchitis), or more than one (e.g. chronic bronchitis and a duodenal ulcer) or none at all (i.e. the 'patient' may not have any disease, but simply have experienced symptoms which raised the possibility of disease). The fact that at one point in time an individual has been confidently allocated to a particular disease category is no guarantee that on another occasion he might not have a different disease, instead or as well, or have recovered completely.

There is no easy solution to any of these problems. Certainly none of them can be eliminated or nullified by a simple change in procedure or strategy. Their most important effect is to throw the whole burden of making diagnosis a viable process onto the quality of the definitions provided for individual diseases. If these are clear cut and unambiguous, diagnosis can still be accurate and reliable, but if they are not, accuracy will deteriorate very rapidly. The reason for this is best illustrated by an analogy. Imagine a naturalist trying to identify a wild flower by comparing it with the illustrations in a flora. His task is greatly simplified by the knowledge that his flower must match one of the illustrations, and only one. If, to begin with, it seems to match two or three of them, or none at all, he is still quite likely with the help of this knowledge to end up with the right answer. But if it were possible that the flower did indeed belong to more than one of the species illustrated in his flora, or none of them, the illustrations would need to be of a very high quality for his accuracy not to be drastically reduced. The definitions we give to individual diseases correspond to the illustrations in this analogy, and need to be of high quality for the same reasons.

Mental illness is a singularly difficult territory in which to achieve this aim. Most psychiatric illnesses are still defined by their syndromes, their typical clinical features, and necessarily so because we know too little of their antecedents to define them at any other level. Many of these clinical features, like depression and anxiety, are graded traits present to varying extents in different people and at different times. Furthermore, few of them are pathognomonic of individual illnesses. In general, it is the overall pattern of symptomatology and its evolution over time that distinguishes one category of illness from another, rather than the presence of key individual symptoms. To put it in technical language, the defining characteristics of psychiatric illnesses are generally both polythetic and inexact.

OPERATIONAL DEFINITIONS

Some years ago, the philosopher Carl Hempel tactfully suggested to an audience of psychiatrists and clinical psychologists interested in problems of diagnosis and classification that they should tackle this situation by developing 'operational definitions' for all the various categories of illness in their nomenclature (Hempel, 1961). This was indeed the only advice any philosopher or scientist could have given. The term operational definition was originally coined by Bridgman (1927) who defined it as follows:

'An operational definition of a scientific term S is a stipulation to the effect

3

that S is to apply to all and only those cases for which performance of test operation T yields the specified outcome O'.

As Hempel himself admitted, in the context of psychiatric diagnosis the term operational has to be interpreted very liberally to include mere observation*. Really, all he is suggesting is that diagnosis S should be applied to all those, and only those, manifesting the characteristic or satisfying the criterion O, subject only to the proviso that O should be 'objective' and 'intersubjectively certifiable' and not simply something experienced intuitively or empathically by the examiner. The crux of the matter is, therefore, how to reduce a range of clinical features, many of which are quantitatively variable and none of which is usually sufficient to establish the diagnosis in question on its own, to a single objective criterion O. This is obviously a difficult and complex task. Indeed much of this book is concerned directly or indirectly with the ways in which it might be achieved. It is only appropriate at this stage to establish two general principles involved. First, individual symptoms or characteristics which are graded traits have to be converted to dichotomous variables by imposing arbitrary cut off points on them, so that the question asked is no longer 'Does the subject exhibit X?', or even 'How much X does he exhibit?', but 'Does he exhibit *this much* X?' Secondly, the traditional polythetic criterion has to be converted to a monothetic one. This can be done quite easily. Instead of saying that the typical features of disease S are A,B,C,D & E and most of these should be present before the diagnosis is made, A,B,C,D, and E must be combined algebraically, so that which combinations satisfy the criterion O and which do not is specified unambiguously. It might be stipulated for instance that any three, or any four, of the five would satisfy O, but other more complex criteria would be equally acceptable provided every possible combination was covered.

*Really it is inappropriate to talk of 'operational' definitions in a setting in which, strictly speaking, no operation is involved. 'Semantic' definition would be a better term, emphasizing that the vital element is the provision of clear cut rules of application (see p. 149). But the term 'operational' has come into widespread use and at this stage it would probably be confusing to try to change it.

# 3 The Issues of Reliability and Validity

## RELIABILITY

Psychiatrists have always realized that their diagnoses did not invariably command the unanimous agreement of their colleagues. However it is only in the last thirty years, and at the prompting of psychologists, that the true importance of this disagreement has been appreciated, and organized attempts made to measure it. Diagnoses are of little value unless useful predictions can be made from them, and if they themselves are subject to disagreement the accuracy of these predictions will inevitably be reduced. If diagnosis A carries a 90 per cent chance of recovery and diagnosis B a 15 per cent chance, the accuracy with which the prospect of recovery can be assessed in an individual patient will largely depend on the accuracy with which A and B can be distinguished from one another. To put the matter as a general principle, the accuracy of the prognostic and therapeutic inferences derived from a diagnosis can never be higher than the accuracy with which, in any given situation, that diagnosis can itself be made; validity can never be higher than reliability and the sporadic assertions to the contrary are based on wishful thinking or sleight-of-hand.

### EARLY STUDIES

The first indications that all was not well appeared in the 1930s. Masserman and Carmichael (1938) followed up a series of 100 inpatients from a university hospital in Chicago and found that a year later a 'major revision in the diagnosis' had to be made in over 40 per cent. To make matters worse, the majority of patients possessed symptoms appropriate to more than one diagnostic category both on initial examination and at follow-up. In the same year, Boisen (1938) demonstrated that the proportion of patients allocated to the different subcategories of schizophrenia in different states, and different hospitals within a single state, varied by a factor of up to ten fold. In Massachusetts, 30 per cent of schizophrenics were catatonic, but in Illinois only 2.7 per cent. In one Illinois hospital, 76 per cent of schizophrenics were hebephrenic but in another only 11 per cent, and so on. Starting about a decade later and continuing throughout

27

the 1950s, numerous studies were mounted, mainly by American workers, with the specific object of testing the reliability of psychiatric diagnosis. In most of these reliability was found to be very low. In an oft-quoted study, Ash (1949) compared the diagnoses given to a series of fifty two men by three psychiatrists after a single joint interview and found that all three made the same specific diagnoses in only 20 per cent of the fifty two, and in 30 per cent all three made different diagnoses. Reviewing a series of eight studies carried out in the following decade Beck (1962) showed that, if organic cases were excluded, none of them achieved an overall agreement rate higher than 42 per cent, at least for the specific diagnosis. Nor were psychologists any more successful than psychiatrists. Goldfarb (1959) studied the diagnostic assessments of four experienced clinical psychologists in Baltimore. Their assessments were based on a Rorschach and a battery of other tests, together with a full psychiatric history, and as cases were assigned to the four quite randomly, each should have generated the same spectrum of diagnoses. In fact, the proportion of cases regarded as psychoneurotic by each varied from 4–48 per cent, and for personality disorders the range was from 22–61 per cent. Similar large differences were obtained when all four were given the same set of 100 clinical reports and test results to report on. Psychoneurotic diagnoses varied from 6–31 per cent and psychophysiologic reactions from 2–16 per cent. When each of them was given the same set of clinical reports and test results again a fortnight later, 40 per cent of the subjects ended up with different diagnoses. Findings such as these produced widespread disillusionment and added further weight to the growing feeling that diagnosis was a futile exercise where mental illness was concerned. Ironically, as Zubin (1967) has pointed out, after being a major but purely academic preoccupation of psychiatrists for several decades, diagnosis fell into disrepute at the very time when the availability of a range of effective and fairly specific therapies was at last providing the exercise with some practical importance.

### Unjustified pessimism

In fact, the pessimism produced by these American studies was never fully justified, for a variety of reasons. In several cases, the setting in which the study was performed weighted the scales against reliability from the beginning. In Ash's study, for instance, two thirds of the subjects were not ill at all and the diagnoses attributed to them were really only ratings of their predominant personality characteristics. Much the same is true of Goldfarb's subjects who were veterans seeking compensation or pensions for service connected disabilities. In other studies, like that of Schmidt and Fonda (1956), some or all of the diagnoses were made by residents who were in these authors' words 'young, foreign trained, inexperienced and psychiatrically naive'. In several others, like that of Hunt, Wittson and Hunt (1953), the diagnoses were made in a military setting in which administrative considerations, like pension entitlements and criteria for discharge from the service, were likely to have been influencing admission and discharge diagnoses in different ways. And in others, like that of Stoer (1964), the study was based selectively on patients who posed diagnostic problems.

Sometimes also, the authors' conclusions were more pessimistic than their findings really justified. Pasamanick, Dinitz and Lefton (1959) compared the diagnoses given to groups of female patients randomly assigned to three different wards in the Columbus Psychiatric Institute over a two year period. Impressed by the variation in the proportion of patients allocated to different diagnostic categories on the three wards they concluded angrily: 'Clinicians, as indicated by these data, may be selectively perceiving and emphasizing only those characteristics and attributes of their patients which are relevant to their own preconceived system of thought. . . they may be so committed to a particular psychiatric school of thought, that the patient's diagnosis and treatment is largely predetermined.' However, as Kreitman (1961) has already pointed out, if one ignores the smallest group of only 48 patients the diagnostic variations between the other wards and psychiatric are all fairly modest, schizophrenia varying from 22–29 per cent, organic disorders from 7–11 per cent, psychoneuroses from 30–45 per cent, character disorders from 12–22 per cent, and so on.

However, by no means all the methodological shortcomings of these early studies were such as to lower reliability. Several must be assumed to have had quite the opposite effect. In some, of which Stoer's study is a particularly glaring example, the diagnoses being compared were not made independently of one another, in others only very broad categories of illness like psychosis and neurosis were distinguished. In Schmidt and Fonda's study, the percentage agreements obtained were inflated by statistical procedures of questionable validity. Frequently it is impossible to tell in which direction the net effect of two or more different defects or limitations in design would be likely to be. As Beck and his colleagues put it, the studies done in this era 'presented certain methodological problems which made the findings inconclusive' (Beck, Ward, Mendelson, Mock & Erbaugh, 1962).

WAYS OF MEASURING RELIABILITY

It is worth distinguishing three different ways of measuring diagnostic reliability, described by Zubin (1967) as observer agreement, frequency agreement and consistency. Measuring observer agreement is the most direct way of assessing reliability, and the most widely used. Each patient is interviewed by two or more diagnosticians either in a single joint interview or in separate interviews a few hours, or at most a few days, apart. The extent of their agreement is then usually expressed as a percentage. Frequency agreement studies are those in which the proportion of patients allocated to individual diagnostic categories by two diagnosticians or teams of diagnosticians are compared in two series of patients whom there is good reason to regard as more or less identical. The attraction of this design is that, provided a setting is available in which this requirement of comparability is met, the study can be executed without any additional interviewing beyond that required for existing service functions. The analysis by Pasamanick, Dinitz and Lefton mentioned above is a typical example. Similar studies, with conflicting findings, have been reported by Mehlman (1952), Wilson and Meyer (1962) and Niswander, Haslerud and Weinstein (1966). Consistency studies are investigations, like that of Masserman and Carmichael, in which the diagnoses given to a group of patients at two widely separated points in time are compared. If the diagnoses are made by different people on the two occasions, as they usually are, this is really a variant of the basic observer agreement design, except that the comparatively long time interval between the two examinations increases the likelihood of disagreements being due to change in the patient, rather than to inconsistency on the part of the diagnosticians. Although the percentage agreement obtained in this setting is almost inevitably lower than in observer agreement studies, it is important for this very reason that such studies should be mounted. A diagnostic system which was unstable from week to week or month to month would be of little use however high agreement between diagnosticians might be at a single point in time.

*Methodological requirements*

Because of the shortcomings of the studies referred to above which he had reviewed, Beck (1962) took the trouble to stipulate what he considered to be the requirements of an adequate reliability study of observer agreement type. All the diagnosticians involved in the study should be experienced, and of comparable experience. They should agree to use a single nomenclature, preferably the most recent version of a standard or national nomenclature, and discuss any ambiguities in it before starting. The duration and setting of their interviews should be kept constant, and likewise the amount of ancillary information provided (psychological test results, information from relatives, etc.). The study should also be independent of routine assessment, to prevent diagnoses being influenced by administrative considerations. Rightly, Beck did not commit himself to a clear preference for either a single joint interview or a pair of separate interviews, though he stressed that if separate interviews were held the interval between them should be short and constant. He also pointed out that the first of these options carries with it the risk of one diagnostician guessing the trend of the other's thoughts from the questions he is asking, and the second the risk of the patient's condition changing in the interval between the two interviews.

It is also possible that the patient might react differently to the second interviewer simply because a repeat interview is a new and different situation from the first.

## THE PHILADELPHIA STUDY

Beck and his colleagues in Philadelphia carried out a reliability study fulfilling these criteria on a series of 153 outpatients (Beck, Ward, Mendelson, Mock and Erbaugh, 1962). Four experienced Board-certified psychiatrists were involved and each patient was seen by two of the four in separate interviews on the same day. The allocation of psychiatrists to patients was random and each interview lasted about an hour. The nomenclature of the original (1952) edition of the *American Psychiatric Association's Diagnostic and Statistical Manual* (DSM–I) was used, augmented by some working definitions drawn up during preliminary discussions. Overall, these workers obtained 54 per cent agreement on the specific diagnosis, compared with the 15–19 per cent agreement that could have been produced by chance alone. This represents a considerable improvement on earlier studies, particularly in view of the fact that their series contained no organic patients and few psychotics. If their alternative diagnoses are also included, agreement rises to 82 per cent. But in spite of this relatively high level of agreement the authors felt bound to conclude that 'there is still a serious question as to whether the rate of agreement for the refined diagnostic categories is high enough for the purposes of research and treatment'.

A valuable and unique feature of this study was that immediately after their interviews each pair of psychiatrists compared their diagnoses and, in the forty patients over whom they disagreed, discussed why they had done so (Ward, Beck, Mendelson, Mock and Erbaugh, 1962). They considered that inconstancy on the part of the patient, either withholding information from one of the two interviewers, or giving a different account in the second interview because of insight gained in the first, was only responsible for 5 per cent of their disagreement. Inconstancy on the part of the interviewer was more important, and estimated to be the cause of 32.5 per cent of the overall disagreement. Included under this heading were differences in interviewing technique causing different items of information to be elicited by the two interviewers, and differences in the diagnostic significance attributed to symptoms which both agreed were present. They attributed most of their disagreement, however, 62.5 per cent of the total, to the inadequacies of the nomenclature they were using. They felt that it required them to make distinctions which were too fine to be practicable, did not provide adequate criteria for distinguishing related syndromes from one another, and, above all, repeatedly presented them with a forced choice between two categories (usually a psychoneurotic disorder and a personality disorder) both of whose requirements had been fulfilled.

THE CHICHESTER STUDY

At much the same time as this, Kreitman was carrying out a similar study on a series of ninety new referrals to the mental health services in Chichester (Kreitman, Sainsbury, Morrissey, Towers and Scrivener, 1961). Each patient was examined independently, first by one of three consultant psychiatrists and then, three to four days later, by one of two psychiatrists from the Medical Research Council unit. Both interviews were unstructured and were held in a variety of different settings (mainly outpatient clinics or the patient's home) and relatives were also seen wherever possible, because it was the aim of the study to stick as closely as possible to ordinary NHS working conditions. Each of the six pairs of psychiatrists involved saw a group of fifteen patients matched with the others for age, sex and social class and, as in the Philadelphia study, working definitions for a number of key terms were agreed upon beforehand. Overall diagnostic agreement, using eleven different diagnostic categories, was 63 per cent, a higher figure than that obtained by Beck and his colleagues, but probably attributable to the higher proportion of psychotic and organic patients in the series.

RELIABILITY IN RESEARCH SITUATIONS

For several years these two studies were widely regarded as an accurate indication of the best diagnostic agreement attainable by experienced psychiatrists, and so they still may be where ordinary working conditions are concerned. But for research purposes at least, considerably higher levels of agreement have now been shown to be feasible. Most of the difficulties produced by variation in interviewing technique from one psychiatrist to another can now be greatly reduced by using standardized interviewing schedules which stipulate not only which topics are to be covered, but which questions are to be asked, and in what order, and how the patients' replies are to be interpreted. Using an early version of his Present State Examination, for instance, Wing and his colleagues held joint interviews with a series of 172 patients and found that sixty nine of the seventy five patients diagnosed as schizophrenic by either rater were so diagnosed by both, a concordance rate of 92 per cent (Wing, Birley, Cooper, Graham and Isaacs, 1967).

A considerable improvement in reliability can also be obtained if all the diagnosticians involved in the study share the same training and orientation, particularly if that training has stressed the importance of observation, rather than inference, and the need for careful definition of terms. In a recent study in which audiences of psychiatrists who had all been trained at the Maudsley Hospital were asked to diagnose an unselected series of newly admitted inpatients after seeing a videotape of a brief interview with each, the average level of inter-rater agreement was 77 per cent in spite of the fact that the interviews lasted a mere 5 minutes and no other information was provided (Kendell, 1973a). Even more impressive was the fact that the average level of agreement between the diagnoses of the videotape raters and the patients' final hospital diagnoses was still 60 per cent (compared with a chance expectation of 25 per cent), in spite of the great disparity in the amount and nature of the information on which the two sets of diagnoses were based, and the very restricted information available to the videotape audiences. As there were good grounds in this study for assuming that this figure of 60 per cent would have been significantly higher had the recorded interviews been longer, the benefits to be derived if all the raters involved in a study have been adequately trained in the same institution are clearly considerable, and well worth striving for in research settings in which diagnostic reliability is all-important.

Another simple means of improving reliability is to rank all the categories recognized, in whichever nomenclature is being used, into a hierarchy, and then stipulate that whenever the defining criteria of more than one category are satisfied the main diagnosis shall be whichever ranks higher in that hierarchy. Beck and his colleagues regarded the problem of double diagnoses, like a neurotic illness in the presence of a personality disorder, as one of the major causes of disagreement in their study, but it ought to be possible to eliminate the problem by means of a simple convention of this kind.

FACTORS INFLUENCING RELIABILITY

The whole of this discussion so far has been based on two crucial assumptions. First that it is meaningful to talk of the reliability of psychiatric diagnosis without regard to the setting, or the range of patients involved, and second, that the percentage agreement between two series of diagnoses is an adequate index of reliability. In fact, neither of these assumptions will bear close examination. The fact that they are implicit in many of the reliability studies referred to here is an important reason why this quite extensive literature provides comparatively little useful information.

*Variation between diagnostic categories*

There is a great deal of evidence that some individual diagnoses are considerably more reliable than others. To quote three examples: Norris (1959) studied a cohort of over 6,000 patients admitted to a number of area mental hospitals in London from a psychiatric observation ward and found that, although concordance between the mental hospital and observation ward diagnoses was 68–70 per cent for schizophrenia, manic depressive psychosis and mental deficiency, for paranoid psychoses and cerebrovascular psychosis it was only 29 per cent. Kreitman and his colleagues in their Chichester study obtained 75 per cent agreement for organic diagnoses and 61 per cent for functional psychoses, but only 28 per cent agreement for neurotic disorders (Kreitman *et al*, 1961). Sandifer, Pettus and Quade (1964) in North Carolina, obtained 74 per cent agreement for a diagnosis of schizophrenia and 73 per cent for mental deficiency, but only 26 per cent for involutional psychotic reaction and 22 per cent for psychotic depressive reaction. [This was in a setting in which ten psychiatrists sitting as a group interviewed and diagnosed a series of ninety one patients.] In general, organic states produce higher concordance rates than functional ones, and psychoses higher concordance rates than neuroses or personality disorders. This means that global reliability is bound to vary considerably with the diagnostic composition of the population being examined, and that inpatient populations, with their relatively high proportion of psychotic patients, will generally produce higher concordance rates than outpatient series composed mainly of neurotic states.

The most obvious way of coping with this problem is to provide separate percentage agreement values for each diagnostic category or group of categories, either alongside or instead of the overall value. But even this does not really solve the problem because the reliability with which any individual category is recognized depends very much on the setting in which this recognition is taking place. For instance, a diagnosis of antisocial psychopathy might well appear to be highly reliable if three or four aggressive men with prison records were encountered in a series composed mainly of chronic schizophrenics and depressed housewives. However, if these same men were encountered in a forensic setting, the reliability of the diagnosis would probably be much lower. It is one thing to distinguish a psychopath from a schizophrenic, but quite another to distinguish him from an ordinary recidivist. Although this may be an extreme example chosen to illustrate the point, comparable situations are almost unavoidable in any reliability study. In general, the category to which any small group of patients who differ from the rest of a series are allocated will appear to be more reliable than it would in other more homogeneous settings. Conversely, the more similar all the members of a reliability study population are to one another, the harder it will be to demonstrate reliable distinctions.

*The Influence of other Variables*

The criteria Beck laid down for the design of an observer agreement reliability study were really those required for measuring the reliability obtainable by experienced psychiatrists under ordinary outpatient working conditions. But, as Kreitman has pointed out, we are also interested, or should be, in how reliability varies from one setting to another. Ideally, we ought to know what reliability can be achieved by experts working under optimal conditions, what by ordinary experienced psychiatrists under normal working conditions, and what by registrars or residents in training. It would also be valuable to know whether diagnoses based on interviews lasting over an hour were more, or less, reliable than those lasting only twenty minutes, and how much difference it makes when information is also obtained from relatives and other ancillary sources. The fact that the overall percentage agreement achieved in any study is heavily dependent on the diagnostic composition of that particular series, and that even the values obtained for individual categories are liable to be influenced by the overall composition of the series, obviously makes it difficult to obtain clear answers to such questions. If one reliability study based on 90 minute interviews produces a higher overall percentage agreement than another based on thirty minute interviews it does not follow that diagnoses based on 90 minute interviews are more reliable than 30 minute ones, unless other factors like the competence of the raters and the diagnostic composition of the patient sample are held constant. In practice, these variables will only be held constant if both studies are part of a single research design. This implies that reliable answers to the questions we are interested in will never be provided by isolated groups of workers carrying out reliability studies of different kinds in different settings independently of one another. Doubtless, some will obtain a higher percentage agreement than others, but it will never be possible to be sure which of the many differences between them is primarily responsible for this percentage difference. Essentially this is the situation which exists at present. Since 1950 thirty or forty studies of the reliability of psychiatric diagnosis have been carried out in many different settings, but between them they convey little useful information beyond demonstrating that reliability is often very low, and generally lower for neuroses and personality disorders than for psychoses and organic states.

*The limitations of percentage agreement as an index of concordance.*

There are other purely statistical reasons why a bald figure for the percentage agreement between two independent series of diagnoses, or the ratio of concordant pairs of diagnoses to all pairs, conveys relatively little useful information. The first and most obvious of these is that the significance of any given percentage depends to a considerable extent on how many categories are in use. 60 per cent agreement, for instance, would mean a lot more across forty categories than it would across four. There are numerous statements in the literature to the effect that agreement was x per cent for the 'broad category' of illness and y per cent for the 'specific diagnosis'. Not only is the number of broad categories and specific diagnoses available not stated, but the meaning of these terms is also left unclear. Is schizophrenia, for example, a specific diagnosis, or does the type of schizophrenia have to be specified as well in order to qualify?

Actually, it is not sufficient just to record the number of categories available, or even the number actually used. If 70 per cent of patients are allocated to a single category, then 49 per cent agreement could be obtained by chance alone, regardless of whether the total number of categories in use was three or thirty. Realizing this, Beck and most subsequent authors have quoted the percentage agreement that could have been produced by chance alone, given the distribution of diagnoses in their study, alongside the percentage agreement they actually obtained. What is really needed, however, is a statistic for measuring concordance which automatically allows for chance agreement and only credits agreement over and above that level. Cohen's Kappa (Cohen, 1960) fulfils this requirement and deserves to be more widely used than it is, though it is only applicable to paired comparisons and not to settings in which a single patient is diagnosed by three or more raters.

(Kappa $(K) = P_o\text{-}P_c/1\text{-}P_c$ where $P_o$ is the observed agreement and $P_c$ the chance agreement. It has a value of $+1.0$ if agreement is perfect, of 0 if agreement is no better than chance, and a negative value if agreement is worse than chance.)

## Serious and trivial disagreements

A final problem which is ignored by most authors is that some diagnostic disagreements are more serious than others. The difference between a diagnosis of simple schizophrenia and one of a schizoid personality disorder is slight and subtle. Yet if different raters attributed these two diagnoses to the same patient, it would rank as a disagreement not only for the specific diagnosis but for the broad category of illness as well, just as if one had diagnosed simple schizophrenia and the other senile dementia. Obviously, the significance of a concordance rate of, say, 60 per cent between two raters will depend very much on whether their disagreements are mainly of the former or the latter type. Foulds (1955) tried to tackle this problem by assigning each possible combination of diagnoses a score on a 7 point agreement scale ranging from 6, perfect agreement, to 0, total disagreement. On such a scale simple schizophrenia v. schizoid personality disorder might score 3 or 4 as a partial agreement, whereas simple schizophrenia v. senile dementia would score 0. Foulds himself found, in a small scale study based on eighteen patients, that the average level of diagnostic agreement between a single pair of psychiatrists was 4. Spitzer and his colleagues in New York have discussed in some detail the inadequacies of concordance rates and contingency coefficients as indices of diagnostic agreement and pointed out that quite high percentage agreement can be obtained by chance alone, even in the presence of a statistically significant $X^2$ value (Spitzer, Cohen, Fleiss and Endicott, 1967). They advocate using $K$ in preference to other more familiar statistics, and show how $K$ can be weighted to allow for differing degrees of disagreement in the way that Foulds suggested. Weighted Kappa ($K_w$) is given by:

$$K_w = 1 - \frac{\Sigma W_{ij} P_{oij}}{\Sigma W_{ij} P_{cij}}$$

where $W_{ij}$ is the weighting assigned to a given pair of diagnoses, represented by the ij cell, $P_{oij}$ the observed proportion with that combination of diagnoses, and $P_{cij}$ the chance proportion with that combination of diagnoses. For diagonal cells, representing identical diagnoses, $W_{ij} = O$, so $K_w$, like $K$ itself, has a value of $+1.0$ if agreement is perfect and of $0$ if it is no better than chance (Cohen, 1968).

## THE PRESENT SITUATION

The reviews of Kreitman (1961) and Beck (1962) have been referred to repeatedly in this discussion. Both gave a balanced and thoughtful account of the studies of the reliability of psychiatric diagnosis done up to that time and their conclusions were broadly in agreement with one another. Essentially, their message was that reliability was low, but not necessarily as low as some earlier studies had suggested, and that a number of ways existed in which it might be raised. Is the situation any different now, a decade later? No large scale observer agreement studies have been mounted since those Kreitman and Beck carried out themselves, perhaps because of a general realization that it was more important to improve reliability than to go on measuring unreliability. However, evidence of the depths to which diagnostic reliability is capable of sinking has continued to accumulate. Katz, Cole and Lowery (1969) presented videotapes of diagnostic interviews with two patients, admittedly chosen because they had so-called 'borderline' symptoms, to audiences of experienced psychiatrists attending meetings of the American Psychiatric Association. The forty four psychiatrists who rated the first videotape made twelve diagnoses between them, and the forty two who rated the second managed to provide fourteen different diagnoses! In each case, these diagnoses were divided more or less evenly between psychosis, neurosis and personality disorder. On the other hand, it is clear both from Katz's work and the similar videotape studies carried out by the US/UK Diagnostic Project (Kendell, Cooper, Gourlay, Copeland, Sharpe and Gurland, 1971) that other patients can command almost unanimous agreement, even between psychiatrists from very varied backgrounds. One of Katz's patients was diagnosed as a schizophrenic by all the forty psychiatrists in the audience and, of the eight videotapes shown to large groups of both American and British psychiatrists by the Diagnostic Project team, two produced almost complete agreement on a diagnosis of schizophrenia and a third unanimous agreement on a diagnosis of depression. Significantly, though, in none of these four examples was there a clear consensus for the type of schizophrenia or depression involved. This adds weight to the evidence of previous studies that it is much harder to make reliable distinctions at this level than it is to distinguish between major syndromes.

*Temerlin's experiment*

The most alarming study to have appeared in recent years is an experiment carried out in Oklahoma by Temerlin (1968). He played an audio tape of an assessment interview with an actor who had been carefully trained to give a convincing account of normality to audiences of psychiatrists and clinical psychologists. Before they heard the recording it was suggested to one audience that the 'patient' or client was psychotic by allowing them to overhear a high prestige figure comment that he was 'a very interesting man because he looked neurotic but actually was quite psychotic'. A second audience was similarly allowed to hear a quite different remark, 'I think this is a very rare person, a perfectly healthy man', and a third audience received no suggestion at all. After hearing the recording, the members of each audience were asked to choose a diagnosis from a list containing ten psychoses, ten neuroses and ten personality types, including 'normal or healthy personality'. All twenty members of the audience given the suggestion of health diagnosed 'normal or healthy personality'. Twelve of the twenty one members of the audience given no suggestion either way also diagnosed normality, but the other nine diagnosed various kinds of neurosis or character disorder. There were ninety five people in the audience given the suggestion that the patient was psychotic, and only eight of these decided that he was mentally healthy. Sixty of them made a diagnosis of neurosis or character disorder and twenty seven a diagnosis of psychosis, usually schizophrenia. When the different professional groups involved were considered separately, it was apparent that the psychiatrists were more suggestible than the clinical psychologists; 60 per cent of them made a diagnosis of psychosis, compared with only 28 per cent of the clinical psychologists, and none regarded the 'patient' as normal. Least suggestible of all, interestingly enough, were a group of clinical psychology students. Significantly, although everyone was asked to describe the 'behavioural basis' for his diagnosis those who diagnosed some form of illness almost invariably justified their diagnoses by inferences rather than by the descriptive statements they had been asked for. It is difficult to imagine a more vivid illustration than this of the dangers of relying on inference rather than direct observation or report, or a more telling indictment of the vague concept of psychosis employed in some circles. Even the pseudo-patients in Rosenhan's study who were diagnosed as schizophrenics by the staffs of the hospitals to which they presented themselves did at least complain of hearing voices (Rosenhan, 1973).

In spite of such findings as these, it can justifiably be claimed that the introduction of structured interviewing techniques, together with the provision of more adequate definitions for both symptoms and diagnoses, and the utilization when necessary of groups of diagnosticians who share a common training, enable psychiatric diagnoses of traditional Kraepelinian type to be made with substantially higher reliability than that obtained by Kreitman and Beck. As the findings of Wing *et al.* (1967) and Kendell (1973a) illustrate, in research settings at least the introduction of such measures can produce acceptable levels of diagnostic concordance.

## The heterogeneity of diagnostic categories

At times the diagnostic categories of psychiatry have been criticized for being heterogeneous as well as unreliable. King (1954), for example, complained that large differences both in symptomatology and in outcome were commonly found between different members of a single category and that 'the difference between two schizophrenics can be as significant as the difference between a normal and a schizophrenic'. As Zigler and Phillips (1961) have pointed out previously, such criticisms are unwarranted. It is characteristic of most biological classifications, including those of disease, to be stratified or tiered. At one level there are a small number of broad heterogeneous categories and at another a larger number of narrower and more homogeneous subcategories. The class of Mammalia is in some respects very heterogeneous but this is in no sense a shortcoming as it is subdivided into numerous genera and species which are more homogeneous. There are considerable advantages in being able to use different levels of generalization for different purposes. The same applies to categories like schizophrenia and neurosis which can also be broken up when appropriate into more homogeneous subcategories.

A more fundamental consideration, though, is that it is meaningless to state that the members of a category are either homogeneous or heterogeneous without stipulating the context. A given group of patients may be homogeneous with respect to overt behaviour, or response to phenothiazines, but highly heterogeneous with respect to mood, or previous occupation. Neither heterogeneity or homogeneity can ever be a global characteristic of any grouping; provided that group is relatively homogeneous with respect to whatever variable is under consideration at the time the grouping is justified, regardless of how diverse its members may be in other respects. It is, of course, important that a category should be relatively homogeneous in at least one chosen respect (which in the context we are concerned with may be either symptomatology, prognosis or aetiology) but this is better regarded as a question of validity than of homogeneity.

## VALIDITY

It has already been stressed that reliability is a means to an end rather than an end in itself. Its importance lies in the fact that it establishes the ceiling for validity; the lower it is the lower validity necessarily becomes. The converse, of course, is not true. Reliability can be high while validity remains trivial and in such a situation high reliability is of very limited value.

Reliability is concerned with the defining characteristics of a class, validity with the correlates of class membership. The more important correlates a given class has, over and above its defining characteristics, the greater the utility of the concept which that class represents. Psychologists have traditionally distinguished four different types of validity, or ways of establishing validity (Zubin, 1967). Briefly, these are:

1. Concurrent validity – the demonstration that independent techniques for arriving at a diagnosis both give the same diagnosis. This might be done by demonstrating that the diagnoses given to a series of patients on the basis of a diagnostic interview by a psychiatrist were the same as those assigned on the basis of responses to a self-report questionnaire like the MMPI. Alternatively, it could be done at a more fundamental level by demonstrating that groupings similar to existing diagnostic categories were produced when patients were sorted into clusters on the basis of their similarity to one another by purely statistical means.

2. Predictive validity – the demonstration that predictions derived from a diagnosis are subsequently borne out by events. These predictions may concern any aspect of prognosis; response to particular therapeutic agents or measures, the development of characteristics or behaviours which were not present at the time the diagnosis was made, mortality, the ability to leave hospital or return to work, and so on. In a sense, this is a question of homogeneity, as useful predictions can usually only be made if most members of the category behave in the same way.

3. Construct validity – the demonstration that aspects of psychopathology which can be measured objectively, like the autonomic arousal of anxiety states or the insomnia of depression, do in fact occur in the presence of diagnoses which assume their presence and not in the presence of those which assume their absence.

4. Content validity – the demonstration that the defining characteristics of a given disorder are indeed enquired into and elicited before that diagnosis is made.

THE PREDICTIVE VALIDITY OF PSYCHIATRIC DIAGNOSES

Of these four, predictive validity is by far the most important. In the last resort all diagnostic concepts stand or fall by the strength of the prognostic and therapeutic implications they embody. The ability to predict what is going to happen, and to alter this course of events if need be, have always been the main functions of medicine. Our modern commitment to elucidating aetiology is really only a strategy for furthering these practical aims rather than an end in itself.

Diagnoses like pulmonary tuberculosis and bronchial carcinoma are useful and valid not because we understand what causes them, indeed there is much about both that we do not understand, but because they enable us to predict fairly accurately what will happen to the patient, and which therapeutic measures will and will not improve that outcome.

How good then is the predictive validity of psychiatric diagnoses? Remarkably few attempts have been made to answer this question directly, though an indirect answer of a sort is implicit in every follow-up study or drug trial involving more than one diagnostic category. As a general rule, whenever two groups of patients belonging to different diagnostic categories are followed up over a period of time, whether or not they are subjected to some specified form of treatment as well, the outcome in the two differs in several statistically significant respects. On the average one group spends longer in hospital, a smaller proportion of its members recover completely, a higher proportion have to be readmitted within a year, and so on. But invariably there is a great deal of overlap between the two, perhaps 65 per cent of one group recover within 3 months but 40 per cent of the other group do likewise. The difference may be highly significant in statistical terms but only rarely is it large enough for confident predictions to be made in individual patients. To complicate the issue further, the diagnostic categories in question usually differ in a number of other respects also. They differ in age, sex and social class distribution, and perhaps in duration of illness as well. Rarely is it formally established that the modest differences in outcome and response to treatment that are observed are due to the diagnostic difference rather than to some combination of these other factors.

Perhaps the most important reason why appropriately designed studies have rarely been carried out is that much of the basic evidence for the validity of our Kraepelinian diagnostic categories accumulated long ago before people began to ask questions about reliability and validity. In the same way that no double blind controlled trial has ever been done to demonstrate the efficacy of digitalis in the treatment of congestive heart failure, because the matter was accepted as proven before controlled trials were ever thought of, so no one has ever set out to prove with matched samples of patients that manic depressive illness remits more frequently than schizophrenia, or that obsessional symptoms are more likely to persist than hysterical ones. If an entirely new classification were to be introduced its validity would undoubtedly have to be established in adequately designed and time consuming studies before it gained acceptance, just as the efficacy of new treatments has to be demonstrated by double blind trials before they supplant existing remedies. But the high suicide rate and relapse rate of manic depressive illness and the tendency to chronicity and progressive deterioration of schizophrenia are too well established, at least in the minds of psychiatrists, for it to be worthwhile at this stage designing a study to demonstrate them.

4

*The Evidence of therapeutic trials*

However, even if there is little direct evidence for, or against, the validity of time-honoured prognostic distinctions such as these, there is a great deal of information relevant to the issue of predictive validity implicit in the results of the numerous therapeutic trials that have been conducted in the last twenty years. These clearly establish the existence of several effective treatments for functional illness – ECT, the phenothiazines, the tricyclic antidepressants, lithium, and other drugs also. It is evident that each of these therapies has a limited sphere of action. ECT is most effective with manic depressive depressions, less effective with schizophrenic or manic illnesses and generally ineffective elsewhere. Phenothiazines are most effective with acute schizophrenic or manic illnesses, less effective with chronic schizophrenic or depressive illnesses and generally ineffective where neurotic syndromes are concerned. Lithium and the anti-depressant drugs show the same sort of pattern: one or two diagnostic categories where their effect is greatest, others where it is weaker but still demonstrable, and others where it is negligible. None of them has an action which is specific to one diagnostic category, and none is consistently effective in more than perhaps two thirds of the members even of that category in which its action is most powerful.

ECT can be used as a convenient illustration of this general situation. Despite the introduction of a wide range of antidepressant drugs, it is still the most effective and rapidly acting treatment for severe depressive illnesses (Medical Research Council, 1965). There is good agreement on the clinical features which correlate with response to ECT, and these correspond quite closely with the clinical features of manic depressive depression (Hobson, 1953; Roberts, 1959; Nyström, 1965). Yet in spite of this, many typical manic depressive depressions fail to respond, while other apparently unrelated syndromes, like catatonic stupor, not infrequently do so. Moreover, it is commonplace for a depressive illness to respond rapidly to ECT on one occasion but fail to do so on a subsequent one, although the patients' symptoms are just the same each time. Finally, a more accurate forecast of the likelihood of response is consistently obtained from scales based directly on symptoms than from the diagnostic category itself (Carney, Roth and Garside, 1965; Nyström, 1965). The situation is similar where each of the drugs referred to above is concerned. Even lithium, which was initially hailed as a specific treatment for the manic phase of manic depressive illness (Johnson, Gershon, Burdock, Floyd and Hekimian, 1971), now appears to be effective against both manic and excited schizoaffective illnesses, and in the latter to affect both schizophrenic and affective symptoms to much the same extent. (Prien, Caffey and Klett, 1972).

The existence of a treatment, like cobalamin for pernicious anaemia or chloroquine for malaria, which was specific for a single diagnostic category, and almost invariably effective on members of that category, would be strong evidence for the validity of that category, but at present no such situation exists in psychiatry. The fact that each of the treatments discussed above is more effective with one category than with others tends to establish the validity of these categories, but the fact that each is effective to some extent in several categories, and inconsistent within all of them, does the reverse.

*Classification by treatment response*

Since the introduction of several effective psychotropic drugs in the 1950's and 60's it has often been suggested that diagnostic categories should be completely recast in terms of treatment response. Instead of schizophrenics, depressives and manics we should have phenothiazine-responders, tricyclic-responders and lithium-responders. At first glance this is an attractive idea. There is widespread dissatisfaction with our existing classification, its categories correspond imperfectly with treatment response, and one of the most important functions of classification is to determine treatment. But there are innumerable snags. Although giving a single treatment to a heterogeneous population, ECT to all depressives for example, generally provides a clear picture of the contrasting profiles of responders and non-responders, the issue becomes much more confused as soon as two or more therapeutic agents are involved.

Because the natural prognosis of most psychiatric syndromes is variable and unpredictable, conclusions about response or non-response can usually only be drawn about populations rather than individuals, and even then only in the context of a controlled trial. Drug A may be more effective than drug B in a limited group of patients, but B may have a broader field of action. C may act faster than D and so be more effective at 3 weeks, but less effective at 3 months. D may be more effective than both A and B when these are given individually, but not when they are given in combination, and so on. Above all, drug response categories are not mutually exclusive in the way that diagnostic categories are. Most tricyclic responders are also ECT responders, and some of them are phenothiazine responders as well. It is also worth remembering that drug response is rarely used as a classificatory principle in other branches of medicine, in spite of the widespread availability of effective drugs, and that because a group of patients all respond to the same drug it by no means follows that their illnesses all have the same aetiology and prognosis as well. As Hamilton once remarked, headaches, bruises and rheumatism all respond to aspirin.

*Diagnosis and choice of treatment*

A rather different aspect of validity to the relationship between diagnosis and the effectiveness of treatment is the relationship between diagnosis and choice of treatment. This was studied by Bannister, Salmon and Lieberman (1964) in a population of a thousand first admissions to a London area mental hospital. After excluding all those who had been treated before admission, who refused treatment, or who had intercurrent physical illnesses, they were able to demonstrate several statistically significant relationships between the diagnosis and the treatment assigned to each. Most of these relationships, however, only held for broad diagnostic categories like schizophrenia or neurosis and nowhere was there anything approaching a one–to–one relationship. In the authors' words, 'the findings are not consistent with the notion that each particular diagnosis leads logically, or habitually, to a particular treatment. It suggests that variables other than diagnosis may be as, or more important than, diagnosis in predicating choice of treatment.' Much the same could be said of the relationship between diagnosis and the effectiveness of treatment.

EVIDENCE DERIVED BY CLUSTER ANALYSIS

An alternative, though less satisfactory, way of establishing the validity of diagnostic categories to demonstrating their predictive value is to demonstrate that they do indeed reflect independent clusters of symptoms, or circumscribed patterns of behaviour. For a remarkably long time after the framework of our present classification was laid down by Kahlbaum and Kraepelin at the beginning of the century, the existence of distinct patterns of this sort was taken for granted in most circles. It was with a sense almost of shock that Masserman and Carmichael (1938) commented on the 'mixed character' of the symptomatology of the hundred patients they studied in Chicago, and the absence of the relationship they had expected to find between current symptoms and pre-psychotic personality. Eighteen years later, Freudenberg and Robertson (1956) carried out a similar study in London and were likewise impressed and dismayed by the enormous overlap of symptoms from one diagnostic category to another, even when symptom ratings and diagnoses were both made by the same psychiatrist. However, this overlap, and the widespread occurrence of patients with symptoms appropriate to more than one diagnostic category, which are now almost universally recognized, do not necessarily imply that Kraepelin's categories are figments of the imagination. It is still possible that the symptom clusters which his disease concepts assume do exist *in re naturae*, albeit in an imperfect state. During the last twenty years elaborate statistical techniques capable, at least in principle, of demonstrating whether they do so or not have been developed and applied to psychiatric data. Using as their raw material comprehensive sets of clinical ratings derived from a large and unselected population of patients, these techniques, known generically as cluster analysis, group the patients in that population on the basis of their overall similarity into a variable number of distinct 'clusters'. Clearly, if the composition of these statistically derived clusters corresponds closely with existing diagnostic categories this constitutes persuasive evidence for the validity of those diagnostic categories.

The principles and limitations of cluster analysis are discussed in some detail in chapter 8. All that need be said here is that many different varieties of cluster analysis have been developed, embodying different assumptions about the statistical properties of the data and utilizing different mathematical definitions of similarity. Because of these differences, different cluster analysis programs may produce different solutions to a single set of data. For example, one program may combine the patients into five clusters, while another may combine the same data into three, of which none, or only one, is recognizably the same as any of the other five. If the original material is in fact composed of fairly distinct groups of patients, this is comparatively unlikely to occur. Conversely, varying solutions of this sort are more likely to occur if there is little innate clustering tendency in the population.

This shortcoming of cluster analysis, the fact that different programs may produce widely differing solutions, was utilized by Everitt and his colleagues to demonstrate the validity of some of the traditional syndromes of psychiatry (Everitt, Gourlay and Kendell, 1971). Clinical ratings derived by structured interviewing methods from two series of 250 patients, one newly admitted to an American state hospital, the other newly admitted to an English area mental hospital, were each subjected to two quite different forms of cluster analysis. From the pool of over 700 items of information available for each patient, seventy key items were chosen and reduced by principal component analysis to ten orthogonal factors prior to the clustering procedure. In this way, four separate cluster analyses were performed on the American and British data separately by each of the two different methods. All four of these analyses produced separate clusters clearly identifiable with the manic and depressive phases of manic-depressive illness, with acute paranoid schizophrenia, and with chronic or residual schizophrenia. The manic and paranoid schizophrenic clusters were particularly clearly defined, and the chronic schizophrenic cluster the least well defined. The fact that substantially the same groups of patients were picked out by both programs from both the American and the British series is persuasive evidence that these diagnostic categories do reflect natural groupings. It is worth noting, though, that other diagnostic groups like depressive neuroses, personality disorders and alcoholism showed no tendency to form distinct clusters in any of the four analyses, in spite of being well represented in the original material.

A rather similar study has been reported by Overall (1971). A consecutive series of 350 consecutive admissions to the inpatient service of a university hospital in Texas was rated on the Factor Construct Rating Scale (FCRS), a set of seventeen 7 point scales, similar to the more well known Brief Psychiatric Rating Scale, concerned with current symptomatology and behaviour. These ratings were subjected to a Q-type factor analysis (see chapter 8) in order to identify and delineate groups of patients with similar patterns of symptoms. In fact, the data were divided randomly into seven groups of fifty patients and the analysis carried out on each of these separately. The four clusters which were accepted from each of these seven solutions were then used as the basis for a second (higher order) analysis which produced five clusters identified by Overall as 'Depression', 'Thinking Disturbance', 'Extrapunitiveness', 'Neuroticism' and 'Agitation Excitement'. The importance of this rather complicated two-stage procedure is that only clusters which had been generated in at least four of the original seven analyses were accepted in the final solution, thereby providing some sort of guarantee that they were genuine and not mere artefacts. FCRS ratings were then obtained for a further, much larger, series of 1032 patients admitted to the same inpatient unit (Overall, Henry and Markett, 1972). Each was allocated, on the basis of a normalized vector product criterion of similarity, to one of these five clusters and the resulting allocations compared with the routine clinical diagnoses given to those same patients. There was a close relationship between the two. Most patients allocated to the depression cluster had clinical diagnoses of depression and most of those allocated to the thinking disturbance cluster had clinical diagnoses either of schizophrenia or of an organic state. Those assigned to the extrapunitiveness cluster tended to receive clinical diagnoses of psychopathy, those assigned to the neuroticism cluster to receive clinical diagnoses of psychoneurosis and those to the agitation/excitement cluster to receive clinical diagnoses of mania.

Although the authors' main aim was to validate their five empirically derived clusters, and they drew attention to several significant relationships between these and a variety of social variables and treatment assignations to that end, their results can also be regarded as a validation of the corresponding clinical categories. Although the titles they gave them were different the patient groupings Overall obtained were substantially the same as the traditional clinical groupings of depression, schizophrenia, psychopathy, psychoneurosis and mania. It could be argued, of course, that in both these cases, Overall's study and Everitt's, the close correspondence between the clusters that were obtained and traditional diagnostic groupings was produced by 'halo' effects; that in each case the raters' perception of patients' symptoms was influenced and moulded by the fact that they expected to encounter particular combinations of symptoms, and not others (Thorndike, 1920). This is an important possibility where Overall's study is concerned as his FCRS ratings were made by residents on the basis of routine unstandardized interviews conducted some time beforehand. It is a less convincing explanation of Everitt's findings as his data were derived from structured interviews carried out by a team of trained research workers.

In summary, evidence for the validity of the traditional diagnostic categories of psychiatry is of three different kinds. Evidence that different diagnostic categories respond differently to a variety of therapeutic measures and have different short and long term prognoses, evidence that diagnostic and therapeutic assignments are related, albeit imperfectly, and statistical evidence that some major categories do reflect genuine symptom clusters. Taken as a whole, this evidence is somewhat meagre, but it is by no means non existent at least where the functional psychoses are concerned.

VALIDITY AND USEFULNESS

The question of validity is closely bound up with that of usefulness. As we have seen, several alternative ways of establishing validity are recognized but the only one of these which also demonstrates that the categories in question have some practical utility is the demonstration that useful predictions can be derived from them. Although the validity of categories like mania, schizophrenia and depression may be demonstrated fairly convincingly by cluster analysis, their usefulness is not enhanced by such evidence. This can only be achieved by demonstrating that they carry different prognoses and respond differently to different therapeutic agents. The greater such prognostic differences are, the more useful the classification. By the same token, as long as these prognostic differences remain as weak as most are at present, the validity and usefulness of our symptom based classification will continue to be questioned.

CLASSIFICATIONS NOT BASED ON SYMPTOMS

There have, in fact, been innumerable suggestions in the last forty years that classification on the basis of symptoms should be abandoned and replaced by an entirely new classification based on data of quite a different kind. It has, for example, been suggested that psychiatric symptoms should be replaced by scores on cognitive or other psychological tests (King, 1954; Frank, 1969); by relationship patterns or styles of interpersonal behaviour (Leary and Coffey, 1955); by social role functioning and social attitudes (Clausen, 1971); by a comprehensive analysis of all behaviour in a wide range of situations (Kanfer and Saslow, 1965); and, most frequently of all, that they should be replaced by psychodynamic defence mechanisms. Almost invariably such suggestions reflect the author's own sphere of interest. With monotonous predictability, clinical psychologists suggest cognitive test results, behaviour therapists suggest total behavioural analysis and psychoanalysts suggest psychodynamic mechanisms. But almost never has any serious attempt been made to develop, test and use an alternative classification on any of these bases. The suggestion is made and the advantages of the innovation emphasized, but it is left to others to implement it. The would-be innovator either lacks the courage of his convictions, or is daunted by the enormity of the task which he has set himself. One may suspect that a classification based on psychodynamic defence mechanisms would be hamstrung by the low reliability common to all inferential judgements, that one based on cognitive test results would yield even fewer useful prognostic distinctions that we have now, and that one based on an analysis of the patient's total behavioural repertoire would simply prove impracticable, but one can do no more than suspect these things because classifications on these bases have never progressed beyond the stage of advocacy. The plain reason why psychiatrists continue to use their traditional symptom-based classification in spite of its low reliability and limited validity is that, as things stand, there is no alternative.

The question of whether the relationship between one patient and another is better expressed by a set of categories or by a set of dimensions has not been raised here, partly because it is discussed in detail in chapter 9 and partly because it is an independent issue. Whether symptoms, or cognitive test results, or psychodynamic mechanisms, or some combination of all three, is chosen as the most appropriate basis for classification both options, a typology or a dimensional system, are still available.

# 4 Diagnosis as a Practical Decision-Making Process

Although a great deal has been said and written about the logical status of diagnoses, and their reliability has been measured and questioned many times, surprisingly little interest has been taken in the practical aspects of diagnosis as a decision-making process. In the 1950's when diagnosis and assessment procedures in general were the main professional concern of clinical psychologists, a considerable literature was generated by them on such matters as the contribution of individual cognitive or projective tests to various tests batteries, the difference between the diagnostic assessments of experienced and inexperienced psychologists, and the difference between assessments made by those who administered the tests and those made by others who were simply given the results to interpret. But as the diagnoses with which this work was concerned were almost exclusively based on test results – cognitive, projective, preceptual or motor – often without the patient even being seen by the diagnostician, the relevance of their findings to the traditional medical method of making a diagnosis by taking a history and examining the mental state is questionable. Even in well designed studies yielding unambiguous results, like that of Kostlan (1954), it is difficult for psychiatrists to draw valid inferences about their own diagnostic behaviour, beyond learning that psychometric test results in general, and projective tests in particular, are of little real value in most situations.

In recent years a few studies have been published in which psychiatrists and other physicians have, for the first time, examined their own diagnostic activities in specially designed experimental situations. The results of these experiments are interesting and instructive, and worth describing in some detail in spite of the doubts that must exist about the validity of drawing conclusions about diagnostic behaviour in real life from behaviour in essentially artificial situations.

The situation in which psychiatric diagnoses are most commonly made is one in which a clinician, armed with a variable amount of background information, like the patient's age and occupation and source of referral, holds a free-ranging interview with the patient, lasting anything from twenty minutes to an hour or more. In this interview he seeks to establish a diagnosis by asking the patient first about his current symptoms and difficulties and then about an ever widening circle of other experiences and events, past and present. If one considers this paradigm situation for a few minutes a number of questions immediately spring to mind:

QUESTIONS TO BE ANSWERED

1. What kinds of information does the clinician use to arrive at a diagnosis, and are some types of information consistently more valuable than others?
2. Can one distinguish distinct styles of gathering information and of reasoning from this information, and are some of these superior to others?
3. What is the role of experience and other personal characteristics in determining the variation in accuracy and economy with which clinicians arrive at diagnoses?
4. How long does it usually take an interviewer to reach a confident diagnosis, and at what stage in a diagnostic interview are the crucial decisions usually made?
5. Are some diagnoses consistently easier to make than others, and if so, why?

A convenient way of describing the little we know about the way in which psychiatric diagnoses are made, and the results of the experimental studies referred to above, is to consider each of these five questions in turn.

*The type of information used*

It has been demonstrated in several different settings that there is no simple relationship between a patient's symptoms and the diagnosis assigned to him even when the same clinicians are responsible for both. (Wittenborn, Holzberg and Simon, 1953; Freudenberg and Robertson, 1956; Nathan, Gould, Zare and Roth, 1969). Although in theory diagnosis is based on symptomatology, and consistent, albeit modest, symptomatic differences can be demonstrated between populations drawn from different diagnostic categories, attempts to define the exact relationship between the two in ordinary clinical practice have usually ended in exasperation or bafflement. As both a cause and an effect of this imperfect relationship between symptoms and diagnosis there is considerable variation in the type and quantity of the information different psychiatrists try to obtain before making a diagnosis. Some concentrate mainly on the patient's current mental state or some particular aspect of this, his overt behaviour in the interview for instance, or the degree of insight he shows into the origins of his symptoms. Others are much more concerned with his personality as a whole, his constitutional endowment, his success in coping with life's demands and his habitual ways of reacting to stress. Others focus on the situation in which his symptoms developed and the reasons why this was so stressful to him. Many of these differences can be related to different conceptions of the nature of mental illness, or to the demands of the setting in which the psychiatrist is operating, so it is not always meaningful to ask which approach is best, or to attempt to choose experimentally between one approach and another. Even allowing for such problems, the fact remains that most psychiatrists attempt to collect quite a lot of information of varying kinds before making a diagnosis, and do so without any real knowledge of which types of information are most valuable, and why. The content of the diagnostic interview is determined by a blend of practical experience and inherited tradition and depends on these, faute de mieux, for its justification.

The results of an ingenious study by Gauron and Dickinson (1966a) in Iowa suggest that, as one might expect, there is considerable variation in the diagnostic usefulness of the various items of information psychiatrists seek to acquire in diagnostic interviews. The results of this study also suggest that psychiatrists have little idea which are the most useful items and which the least. What Gauron and Dickinson did was this. They analysed the case histories of three patients and artificially divided each of them into thirty six different information categories – childhood history, projective test results, reason for referral, previous personality, and so on. A group of twelve psychiatrists were then allowed to ask for these units of information, one at a time, in whatever order they liked. After receiving each new piece of information they were required to suggest one or more diagnoses, together with an estimate of the probability of its being correct. This process continued until they either had all thirty six units of information, or were confident in their final diagnosis. At the end the twelve participants were asked to list in order, for each of the three patients, the five pieces of information they felt had been most important in determining their final diagnosis. By recording which items of information had first suggested his three final diagnoses to each participant, and which had increased the probability ratings of these at each stage thereafter, the authors were able to calculate an actual order of importance for the thirty six items, to compare with the perceived order. Not unexpectedly, 'reason for referral' came first by a wide margin in both lists, but thereafter there was little or no relationship between the two and the rank order correlation between them was too small to be statistically significant.

Traditionally, the mental state and the history have always been regarded as the two basic components of the diagnostic interview, the latter sometimes being obtained wholly or in part from a relative. Which of these is, or should be, more important and how often relatives or other informants provide crucial information not obtainable from the patient are both questions which have rarely been posed. Simon, Gurland, Fleiss and Sharpe (1971) analysed how frequently, in a series of 400 patients, information elicited from the patient in a semi-structured history interview resulted in the revision of a diagnosis originally based solely on a structured mental state interview and found that changes were uncommon and did not alter the overall distribution of diagnoses. But this is not necessarily evidence of the unimportance of historical data, even in the hands of these particular psychiatrists. Unless elaborate precautions are taken, a variable and often substantial amount of historical information is acquired in the course of any detailed examination of the current mental state, and vice versa, and measures of how often diagnoses are changed are at least partly an index of how willing the diagnostician is to change his mind. However, some confirmation of the primacy of the mental state examination is provided by Gauron and Dickinson's study. Although only six of their thirty six information categories were derived from the mental state, four of these came in the first ten in the perceived order of importance and four in the first eleven in the actual order. Past history categories, on the other hand, did not figure prominently in either list, and the authors comment on their surprise at this finding – 'for all practical purposes, the patient's mental state at the time of evaluation was the major determinant of how he was classified, irrespective of the other information'. It must be appreciated, though, that the relative importance of mental state and history will vary considerably from one type of patient to another, the former generally being more important in psychosis and the latter more important in other diagnoses such as personality disorders. In other types of patients, alcoholics for example, there would probably be little difficulty in demonstrating that information from another informant was often vital for accurate diagnosis.

Several people, including some of their participants, have suggested that the diagnostic situation in Guaron and Dickinson's study was so artificial that the significance of its findings for real life diagnostic interviewing is rather dubious. However, a similar finding, that psychiatrists rely much more on some types of information than others, and are unaware which they are using, emerged from a quite different type of study by the author (Kendell, 1973a). In this experiment, videotapes were made of brief diagnostic interviews, lasting exactly 5 minutes each and concerned mainly with the reason for admission to hospital, with a series of twenty eight unselected psychiatric patients. These were presented to audiences of experienced psychiatrists in three alternative ways, as a videotape (vision and sound), as an audiotape (sound only), and simply as a written transcript. To the author's surprise, the accuracy of the audiences' diagnoses, using the patients' final hospital diagnoses as a criterion, was just as high when they were given only the audiotape or the transcript as when they were shown the full videotape. Moreover, in spite of Gauron and Dickinson's conviction that psychiatrists are not 'comfortable' with their diagnosis unless they are able to see the patient, the same was true of their confidence in their diagnoses. The mean ratings on a five point confidence scale appended to the rater's main diagnosis were just as high for the audiotapes and the transcripts as for the videotapes. As in the Iowa study, participants were required to indicate for each patient which individual items of psychopathology their diagnosis was mainly based upon. Forty four per cent of the items singled out by the videotape audiences as diagnostically important were behavioural ones which were not available to those whose diagnoses were based solely on the transcripts of the interviews. But as the transcript diagnoses were just as accurate, and inspired just as much confidence, as those based on the original videotapes, one is forced to conclude that the behavioural items the videotape raters regarded as important were in fact superfluous. The other implication of this, that psychiatrists rely almost entirely on what the patient says, rather than on the way he behaves, can be used to justify the use of audiotapes or transcripts for research purposes instead of live interviews, and rebuts the argument that to do so involves losing vital information.

*Styles of information gathering and decision making.*

It is well known that some clinicians always ask the same questions in much the same order regardless of the patient's replies, while others are strongly influenced by what the patient says, and by their own developing diagnostic impressions, and vary the questions they ask accordingly. Others appear, at least to the onlooker, to ask questions more or less at random. For convenience, these will be referred to as the 'set order', 'train of thought' and 'haphazard' styles of questioning. How widespread distinct styles of this sort are in practice, what the relative advantages and disadvantages of the 'set order' and 'train of thought' approaches are in different situations, and to what extent interviewers tend to shift from one to another according to the type of patient they are dealing with, are for the most part unanswered questions. It does seem, though, that experienced physicians usually vary their questions with the patient's replies and are hypothesis testing, rather than simply data gathering, from quite an early stage in an assessment interview. The studies of diagnostic behaviour mounted at the Michigan State University suggest that experienced physicians usually formulate a number of alternative diagnoses very early in their interview and spend most of the time thereafter attempting to confirm or refute these hypotheses, rather than starting by systematically gathering data and formulating their diagnosis towards the end (Elstein, Kagan, Shulman, Hiliard and Loupe, 1972). Similar conclusions emerged from a recent study in Leeds of the diagnostic behaviour of surgeons examining patients with abdominal pain (Leaper, Gill, Staniland, Horrocks and de Dombal, 1973). The results of this extensive and carefully designed investigation demonstrated that inexperienced house surgeons tended to have an inflexible, stereotyped approach, the 'set order' style, whereas more experienced registrars and consultants followed a recognizable train of thought, and as a result asked fewer questions and achieved considerably higher efficiency. The investigators also found, though, that diagnostic styles varied considerably from patient to patient as well as from doctor to doctor.

Such studies as these have obvious relevance to the controversy over the relative merits of structured interviews, in which the sequence of questions is predetermined, and unstructured ones in which the interviewer is free to follow his own train of thought. For research purposes the advantages of the former are clear cut. Reliability is increased and the set format ensures that the same range of topics is covered in every patient. But in ordinary clinical situations, in which the emphasis is on the patient as an individual rather than as a member of a population, these issues are relatively unimportant. What matters is to elucidate the patient's key symptoms and formulate a diagnosis as easily and as quickly as possible. Even so, comparisons between structured and unstructured diagnostic interviews suggest that the balance of advantages and disadvantages does not necessarily lie with the latter (e.g. Saghir, 1971).

In the experiment described in the previous section, Gauron and Dickinson (1966b) described observing several distinct styles of information gathering corresponding more or less to the 'set order', 'train of thought' and 'haphazard' stereotypes but they also comment that many of their subjects adopted different strategies with different patients, and one suspects from their description that the clearly defined styles they describe owe as much to reasoned expectation as to actual observation. They described a number of different styles of decision making as well, though these too were prone to change from one patient to the next. Some of their raters started by considering several different diagnoses, each at a low level of probability, and systematically eliminated these one after the other until only one remained. Others kept changing the diagnosis they considered most probable, apparently because they were over influenced by the information they had acquired most recently and forgot the earlier items which had already led them to discard that diagnosis. A third type, to which they drew particular attention, was exemplified by a number of their raters who committed themselves to a single diagnosis at an early stage on insufficient evidence, and then stuck tenaciously to this even in the face of information strongly indicative of some other condition. For this reason in the 5 minute videotape study also described in the previous section, the author looked for evidence of this 'premature decision' style by examining how often, and under what conditions, raters made different diagnoses at the end of the interview from those they had made after the first 2 minutes. In fact, none of the twenty eight psychiatrists involved in that study stood out as particularly unwilling, or particularly prone, to change his mind, and there was no detectable tendency for the group as a whole to be reluctant to change their initial diagnoses if appropriate evidence emerged later on in the interview. Doubtless, the phenomenon Gauron and Dickinson described does occur, but on this evidence it does not appear to be a serious problem amongst trained psychiatrists.

*The role of experience and other personal characteristics*

In most settings, and certainly in professional examinations, it is taken for granted that the diagnoses of experienced psychiatrists are more likely to be correct than those of their junior colleagues. To some extent this is inevitable, if only because any training process involves learning to imitate the behaviour and reproduce the judgements of more experienced teachers. But what the crucial differences are between experienced and inexperienced diagnosticians, once the latter are sufficiently experienced to be familiar with the relevant diagnostic stereotypes, and at what stage increased experience ceases to be accompanied by any demonstrable increase in diagnostic accuracy, are largely matters for conjecture. The differences in interviewing style between experienced and inexperienced surgeons observed by Leaper and his colleagues have already been described. In their experiment Gauron and Dickinson were likewise impressed by a number of differences between first year residents and staff psychiatrists in spite of the small numbers of each involved. The former were more likely to make confident diagnoses too early on inadequate evidence, to revert to a diagnosis which they had previously excluded, and to rely relatively exclusively on mental state findings and psychological test results. The latter were more confident in their ability to make an accurate diagnosis without seeing the patient, were both more consistent and more flexible in the way in which they obtained information, and made relatively greater use of historical data.

In the 5 minute videotape study described previously the author examined the relationships between four characteristics of the twenty one psychiatrists who had provided the bulk of the ratings – their length of experience of psychiatry, their diagnostic accuracy (defined as the percentage agreement between their diagnoses and the patients' final hospital diagnoses), their diagnostic confidence (defined as the average rating on a 5 point confidence scale given by the rater to his own diagnoses), and their symptom threshold (defined as the average number of symptoms rated per patient.) None of the six correlations between these four variables even approached statistical significance. The most experienced psychiatrists were no more confident and no more accurate than their more junior colleagues, and those who were most confident in the accuracy of their diagnoses were in fact no more accurate than anyone else. In interpreting these findings, particularly the absence of any relationship between diagnostic accuracy and length of experience, it is important to appreciate that all the psychiatrists involved in the study had had a minimum of four year's experience. Presumably if others with, say, only a year's experience had been included a significant positive correlation would have emerged. This negative finding does suggest though that, after four years of training, whatever other professional skills may continue to develop, diagnostic acumen does not, at least to any measurable extent.

## *The importance of the first few minutes*

Although a diagnostic interview may frequently last for an hour or more there are many indications that the interviewer's final diagnosis is often formulated at a very early stage. The finding of the Michigan studies that most of a physician's assessment interview is spent testing hypotheses that have been formulated in the first few minutes has already been referred to and the same seems to occur in psychiatry. Sandifer, Hordern and Green (1970) showed films of diagnostic interviews with thirty unselected patients, recently admitted to a public mental hospital in North Carolina, to audiences of between fourteen and eighteen psychiatrists drawn from both North Carolina and Britain. The films ran for an average of 25 minutes but were interrupted at regular intervals and the raters asked to record their diagnostic impressions verbatim on a tape recorder and complete a symptom check list at each of these stopping points. It transpired that fully half the symptoms elicited at any stage were reported within the first 3 minutes of these interviews, and that the raters' preferred diagnoses after the first 3 minutes were the same as their final diagnoses three times out of four. Gauron and Dickinson (1969) have also commented on the ease and rapidity with which diagnostic impressions are formed by psychiatrists watching a filmed interview, 'very often within the first 30 to 60 seconds'.

The author's videotape study provides further evidence of the crucial role of the early minutes of the interview. In each of the twenty eight 5 minute interviews used in this experiment, the patient was asked the same fairly standard questions about why he was entering hospital, what had been troubling him recently, in what way he was different from his normal self, and whether he regarded himself as ill. In every rating session the videotapes were stopped and the audience required to make a diagnosis after the first 2 minutes, and then played through to the end and a further diagnosis required. These '2 minute' and '5 minute' diagnoses were then compared with the patients' final hospital diagnoses, which were based on extensive information both from the patient and other informants, and the notes of previous admissions also in many cases. In spite of the great disparity in the amount of information available to the videotape raters and the clinicians responsible for the hospital diagnoses, there was 48 per cent agreement between the two even at 2 minutes, and 60 per cent agreement at 5 minutes. As formal studies of the reliability of psychiatric diagnosis rarely achieve more than 60–65 per cent agreement between independent diagnoses based on full length interviews, it is clear that most of the diagnostically important information in a clinical interview is available in the first few minutes and that a high proportion of diagnoses are, or can be, made correctly at that stage.

There are obviously both advantages and dangers in this situation. The main advantage is one of economy. If an accurate diagnosis can be established after only 5 or 10 minutes in a high proportion of patients so much the better, particularly as there are many situations even in affluent countries where that is all the time that is available. The other side of the coin is a matter of concern to the research worker rather than the clinician. If an interviewer reaches a confident diagnosis in the early stages of a long interview, all the ratings and decisions he makes from that time on are likely to be biased by the 'halo effects' of that initial global judgement (Guildford, 1954). At first sight the duration of the traditional diagnostic interview is called in question by these findings, for if an accurate diagnosis can generally be made after 5 or 10 minutes what is the point of going on longer? The answer is that, at least in ordinary clinical practice, the so-called diagnostic interview is not concerned only, or even mainly, with establishing a diagnosis in the restricted sense used here. The interviewer wants to find out what sort of person his patient is, why he has become ill, whether he has been ill before and what treatment he had then, and so on, and it is these other functions which occupy most of the time. But in research settings in which establishing a diagnosis is the sole function of an interview, there are strong grounds for reducing its length, and also for relying mainly or entirely on non-behavioural data in view of the evidence that behavioural ratings are both less valuable (*vide supra*), and also less reliable than those based on the patient's replies to questions (Kendell, Everitt, Cooper, Sartorius and David, 1968; World Health Organization, 1973a).

*Easy and difficult diagnoses*

It is a matter of common experience that some patients can be allocated almost immediately, and with high inter-rater agreement, to the appropriate diagnostic category, while others defy easy allocation no matter how long they are studied and how much information is collected. Why is this so, and what are the distinguishing characteristics of 'easy' and 'difficult' patients?

The difference is determined partly by the diagnostic category to which the patient belongs. In general 'easy' diagnoses are also reliable ones and, as we have already seen in chapter 3, there are fairly consistent differences in the relative reliability of different categories. The reliability of psychoses is generally higher than that of neurotic states or personality disorders, that of organic psychoses is higher than that of functional psychoses, and that of broad syndromes like schizophrenia and depression is invariably higher than that of specific diagnoses like hebephrenia or anti-social personality disorder. These differences are determined largely by how well the defining characteristics of

5

individual categories are specified, and distinguished from those of other related syndromes. If a syndrome possesses pathognomonic features, like the 'first rank' symptoms of schizophrenia or the morbid attitudes to food and body image of anorexia nervosa, reliability is likely to be high. If, on the other hand, a diagnosis does not possess any features which are specific to itself, and is therefore defined mainly by the absence of the specific features of other syndromes, its reliability is likely to be low, partly because it almost inevitably comes to function as a convenient 'rag bag' for a heterogeneous assortment of patients who do not belong elsewhere.

But this is only part of the explanation because there are big differences in ease of diagnosis between members of the same diagnostic category. It is obvious within a few minutes that some patients are schizophrenic. In others, the same diagnosis takes a long time to establish and still remains a matter of dispute. In most cases the explanation of such differences lies in the degree of similarity between the individual patient's symptoms and those of the textbook description or stereotype of the diagnosis in question. If the two are almost identical the target is hit on the bull's-eye and the diagnosis is easy. But if there is only a degree of resemblance, the target is hit, if at all, only on one of its outer rings and it becomes a harder and less certain task to decide which of several alternative bull's-eyes the shot is nearest to.

Other factors also influence the situation. Patients vary in the accessibility of their symptomatology. Some give unambiguous answers to questions and do not conceal, deny, exaggerate or misinterpret their symptoms. Others are suspicious, evasive, mute or incoherent. The setting in which diagnosis takes place is also relevant. It is easier to identify an aggressive young man with a criminal record as a psychopath when he is encountered in an outpatient clinic attended mainly by depressed housewives than when he is encountered in prison in the company of other recidivists.

Several of these points are illustrated by the findings of the 5 minute videotape study referred to previously. For five of the twenty eight patients in that study every member of an audience of between seven and eleven experienced psychiatrists diagnosed some form of depressive illness, for two others everyone diagnosed schizophrenia and for one everyone diagnosed alcoholism. However, in none of these eight patients was there agreement on the type of depression, schizophrenia or alcoholism involved, emphasizing how much harder it is for psychiatrists to reach agreement on specific diagnoses than on broad syndromes. In fact, only three of the twenty eight patients in the series were given the same specific diagnosis, i.e. the same ICD 4 digit category, by every rater. One of these had a manic illness, one had anorexia nervosa and the other was a transvestite, all syndromes based on well defined symptoms that are rarely encountered in other conditions. In the whole series, fifty three out of a total of 252 5-minute diagnoses were given a confidence rating of 1, indicating that the rater regarded the clinical findings as pathognomonic of the specific diagnosis in question. Twenty two of these fifty three were psychotic states, whereas only seven were neurotic conditions personality disorders, demonstrating how poorly defined the latter are compared with the functional psychoses. (The remaining twenty-four diagnoses were accounted for by three patients with alcoholism, anorexia nervosa and transvestism respectively.)

# 5 Disease Entities in Psychiatry

THE PLATONIC AND HIPPOCRATIC TRADITIONS

The historical evolution of our concept of disease was referred to in chapter 2, but at that time no mention was made of one particularly important aspect of that development – the recurring conflict between the Platonic and Hippocratic traditions. The origins and fluctuating fortunes of these two schools have been described in some detail by Cohen (1943) and more recently by Engle (1963). Essentially, it is a philosophical rather than a purely medical controversy, and one with an ancient lineage, but from the earliest times it has had a profound influence on assumptions about the nature of disease.

Plato maintained that unchangeable reality resided in universal ideas rather than in the individual objects of our senses, which he regarded as relative, imperfect and subject to the Heraclitean flux. Aristotle, on the other hand, had little sympathy with the element of mysticism in this 'doctrine of universals'. His interest was always fixed firmly on the world of his senses and the individual objects and events which made up that world. These two antagonistic yet complementary philosophical attitudes were reflected by the two great schools of medicine of the greek world. The Hippocratic school at Cos was essentially Aristotelian in outlook and its main interest and achievement lay in a meticulous study of the varied manifestations and natural history of disease in individual patients. The rival school at Cnidos had a Platonic orientation and its primary interest was in the universals of medicine – diagnosis and the classification of diseases. Its members are said, for example, to have distinguished seven different diseases of the bile and twelve of the bladder.

These contrasting attitudes have existed side by side ever since, both in medicine and in other branches of learning, though they have often been disguised by a bewildering variety of banners and slogans, Platonic v. Hippocratic, Cnidian v. Coan, ontological v. biographical, realist v. nominalist, rationalist v. empirical, conventional v. naturalistic, and so forth. As Cohen (1943) says: 'The names are of little importance. The two notions varying a little in content and occasionally overlapping have persisted, the dominance of

60

the one or the other at different epochs reflecting either the philosophy of the time or the influence and teaching of outstanding personalities.'

## Sydenham and Linnaeus

In the 17th and 18th centuries the Platonic school was in the ascendant. The English physician Thomas Sydenham, in spite of being a brilliant clinical observer in the finest Hippocratic tradition, insisted that diseases possessed a uniform presentation, and by implication an independent existence, analogous in every way to that of botanical species:

'Nature, in the production of disease, is uniform and consistent; so much so, that for the same disease in different persons the symptoms are for the most part the same; and the self-same phenomena that you would observe in the sickness of a Socrates you would observe in the sickness of a simpleton.'

In an oft-repeated passage he emphasized that diseases 'were to be reduced to certain and determinate kinds with the same exactness as we see it done by botanic writers in their treatises of plants', and that this could be done by virtue of 'certain distinguishing signs which nature has particularly affixed to every species'. This firmly held belief in the existence of disease entities, and the zeal to search for them, was shared by most of Sydenham's contemporaries and was powerfully reinforced for his successors by the publication, in 1735, of Linnaeus' comprehensive taxonomy of plant species, the *Systema Naturae*. Even more influential than Linnaeus' actual classification was his belief in the fixity and immutability of his species – 'species tot sunt diversae quot diversae formae ab initio sunt creatae'. Inspired by his fellow botanist's example, the French physician Boissier de Sauvages published in 1763 his *Nosologia Methodica Sistems Morborum* in which 2,400 species of disease were solemnly listed, neatly divided into classes, orders and genera. A few years later Cullen and Linnaeus himself elaborated this even further.

## Koch and Virchow

In the latter half of the eighteenth century and the first half of the nineteenth the pendulum swung the other way. Rousseau expressed the new spirit very well with his remark that 'Il n'y a pas de maladie, il n'y a que des malades' (There are no illnesses, only sick people), and influential physicians like Broussais and Magendie in France and Muller in Germany regarded disease as a quantitative rather than a qualitative deviation from normality. In 1847, the young Virchow stated boldly that 'Diseases have no independent or isolated existence. . . .they are only the manifestations of life processes under altered conditions.' (Later on he was to repudiate this opinion, but not for the first or the last time youth was right.) Broussais went even further and derided any attempt to delineate syndromes and the typical course of each. 'Those groups of symptoms', he wrote, 'which are given out as diseases are metaphysical distractions which by no means represent a constant unchangeable morbid condition. . . . They are factitious entities.' But the discoveries of Koch and Pasteur in the latter half of the nineteenth century rendered such views untenable. As, one by one, each of the infections that had dominated the practice of medicine for centuries, tuberculosis, syphilis, typhoid, even cholera and malaria, was shown to be due to the presence of a specific microorganism, the tacit assumption that all other diseases were also discrete entities, each with its own distinct cause and distinctive symptoms, became almost irresistible, as Virchow's volte face illustrates. Indeed much of the power and the prestige of 20th century medicine has been based on, and has in turn reinforced, the rationalist assumptions of Koch and Virchow. Cohen, writing in the 1940s, was keenly aware that most of his contemporaries accepted these assumptions without question and a decade later the controversy between Platt and Pickering over the nature of essential hypertension illustrated how difficult it was even then to challenge them. (Oldham, Pickering, Fraser Roberts and Sowry, 1960).

This brief description of the ebb and flow of fortune attending the Platonic and Hippocratic traditions certainly gives too clear cut an impression of the historical relationship between the two. For one thing, the two have always coexisted, and need to do so as Engle has pointed out. But it does illustrate the essential fact that there has been a repeated cyclical change in the balance between them, with first one and then the other becoming the dominant philosophy of the age. We are now entering an empirical or Hippocratic era once more. We accept for example, that essential hypertension is merely a quantitative deviation from normality and that it is no more likely to have a single discrete cause than crime or poverty. But doubtless the pendulum will swing back once more sooner or later.

### Kraepelin and his contemporaries

Our existing classification in psychiatry was born in a Platonic age. Kahlbaum and Kraepelin were cast in the same mould as Sydenham. Both took it for granted that the variegated and shifting forms of mental illness with which they were confronted, or at least the various forms of madness with which they were primarily concerned, consisted of a finite number of disease entities, each with its own distinct cause, psychological form, outcome, and cerebral pathology. They were also brilliant clinical observers and the syndromes they delineated from the midst of chaos rapidly gained widespread and enduring recognition. But their victory was never complete. Just as fifty years earlier Zeller and Griesinger had scorned all attempts to subdivide what to them was a single unitary psychosis, die Einheitspsychose, so fifty years later Karl Menninger

(1963) was insisting that all mental illness was essentially one condition and schizophrenia merely a convenient term for the more severe forms of it. Even in Kraepelin's own day there were a few discordant voices. Hoche's (1910) tart commentary on Kraepelin's classification and the assumptions underlying it is in the purest Hippocratic tradition, quite unmoved by the spirit of the times:

'It is here that a kind of thought compulsion, a logical and aesthetic necessity, insists that we seek for well-defined, self-contained disease entities, but here as elsewhere, unfortunately, our subjective need is no proof of the reality of that which we desire, no proof that these pure types do, in point of fact actually occur.'

The essence of the dispute between the Platonic and Hippocratic traditions, in psychiatry as in medicine as a whole, has always centred around the concept of disease entities, the former maintaining that such things exist, and bent on identifying them, the latter regarding them as man-made abstractions, at best an irrelevance, at worst a dangerous source of misconceptions distracting us from reality. The true relationship between these two contrasting attitudes, and the justification for each, has often been obscured by the smoke of combat. As Jaspers (1959) observed 'The battle between the two camps has been fought with a good deal of mutual contempt and everyone was convinced of the total fiasco created by the endeavours of the opposite camp. Yet in view of the actual history we may suspect. . . . that both camps were on the track of something valid and could well complement each other instead of wrangling'.

## Jaspers' standpoint

Jaspers went on to analyse the concept of a disease entity held by Kahlbaum and Kraepelin and pointed out that, by assuming that each disease had its own distinct cause, psychological symptoms, course, outcome and cerebral pathology they were in fact assuming that the same classification of patients would result regardless of whether aetiological, psychopathological or neuropathological criteria were used. In fact, as he also points out, no entities fulfilling these exacting criteria have ever been found within the realm of psychiatry. None of the diseases Kraepelin himself described does so. Even general paralysis is defined by purely neurological, histological and aetiological criteria and lacks any characteristic psychopathology.

This conclusion does not drive Jaspers into the empiricist camp, however. In fact his position is a very interesting one. For him the idea of a disease entity 'is an idea in Kant's sense of the word: the concept of an objective which one cannot reach since it is unending; but all the same it indicates the path for fruitful research and supplies a valid point of orientation for particular empirical investigations'. Posing the original question again, whether there are only stages and variants of a single Einheitspsychose or a series of disease entities, he concludes: 'There are neither. The latter view is right in so far that the idea of disease entities has become a fruitful orientation for the investigations of special psychiatry. The former view is right in so far that no actual disease entities exist in scientific psychiatry.' Engle's observation that the practical task of making a diagnosis in an individual patient always involves a 'psychic shuttle' to and fro between the unique individual in one's consulting room and the abstract concept of the disease entity, and involving both as the two poles of the axis, is a different way of attempting the same synthesis.

DISEASE ENTITIES IN CONTEMPORARY MEDICINE

Even though their expectations have not been fulfilled, Kraepelin and his contemporaries were quite clear what they meant by the term disease entity. It was derived from the assumption that each disease had a single discrete cause, not merely a 'necessary' cause but a 'sufficient' cause whose presence invariably produced the disease regardless of what other factors were operating. As this cause was assumed to produce a distinctive clinical picture, with a distinctive course and a distinctive neuropathology also, it was unnecessary to stipulate at which level the illness was being defined. The end result would have been the same regardless. The simplicity of the concept shielded it from ambiguity.

Looking back on these assumptions with the hindsight provided by a lapse of seventy years, they appear very naive. In fact, they were simply a reflection of 19th century determinism. The concept of causality prevailing at that time was based on the assumption that similar causes always produced similar effects, that effects were proportionate to their causes, and that every phenomenon had to have its specific antecedent. In such a milieu as this (interpreted by Cameron (1953) as a reaction against the assumption of previous generations that phenomena in general, and sickness in particular, were the capricious manifestations of magical and transcendental forces), it was almost inevitable that people should assume that each illness had its own specific cause. Initially, events bore out this assumption as first GPI and then pellagra had its cause triumphantly elucidated. But today our view of causality is a very different one. In medicine as in physics, specific causes have given way to complex chains of event sequences in constant interplay with one another. The very idea of 'cause' has become meaningless, other than as a convenient designation for the point in the chain of event sequences at which intervention is most practicable.

*'Disease entity' or useful concept?*

In spite of the fact that its original raison d'etre has long since been abandoned, contemporary writers still make frequent references to 'disease entities', 'valid entities', 'genuine entities' and the like, almost invariably without defining their meaning. Like 'disease' itself, 'entity' has become one of those dangerous terms which is in general use without ever being defined, those who use it fondly assuming that they and everyone else knows its meaning. Sometimes the writer provides evidence to substantiate his claim that a particular syndrome is an entity and thus gives some insight into his meaning. Usually this evidence consists of a demonstration that patients with syndrome A have a significantly different prognosis, or response to some therapeutic agent, from those with a related syndrome B; or that patients exhibiting the two syndromes differ significantly on a range of social variables like age, sex and ethnic background. Evidence of this nature is certainly inadequate for establishing the existence of an entity in Kraepelin's sense. Indeed it is difficult to see what it does establish, beyond illustrating that the syndrome in question differs in important ways from its neighbours, and may therefore be worth distinguishing from them. Another variant is to claim that a syndrome is an entity because it has been demonstrated that the close relatives of patients with that syndrome tend to have the same symptoms themselves (e.g. Robins and Guze, 1970). This may well be evidence that genetic factors are involved, but that is all. The close relatives of those who are very tall or very clever also tend to possess those same characteristics, yet no one concludes from this that great height or high intelligence are entities. One suspects that in all these cases the term 'useful concept' would be more appropriate, and certainly less confusing, than arcane references to undefined entities.

## The criterion of discontinuity

It seems to the present writer that if the term entity is to have any meaning at all in contemporary psychiatry, or in any other branch of medicine, it should imply the existence of a natural boundary or discontinuity between the condition in question and its neighbours. In terms of the familiar aphorism that classification is the art of carving nature at the joints, it should imply that there is indeed a joint there, that one is not sawing through bone.

At present, the majority of psychiatric disorders, psychotic and neurotic, are defined in terms of their clinical symptoms. In Scadding's terminology their 'defining characteristic' is their syndrome (Scadding, 1963). If a psychiatric disorder is to be established as a disease entity on this basis, a natural boundary has therefore to be demonstrated between its symptoms and those of its neighbours. If the putative boundary lies between one syndrome and another this means demonstrating, on an unselected population, that patients with features of both conditions are less common than those with symptoms appropriate only to one or the other. And in the related case where the presumed boundary lies between a syndrome and normality, it means demonstrating that patients with partial or half-fledged symptoms are less common than those who have all or none. Either way the mixed forms, the greys, must be shown to be less common than the pure forms, the blacks and the whites. The mere existence of patients with mixed symptoms is not evidence that the boundary is not a genuine one, any more than the existence of a few hermaphrodites invalidates the distinction between male and female, but such interforms must be relatively infrequent. In graphical terms, this means that the distribution curve of the total population must be bimodal rather than unimodal.

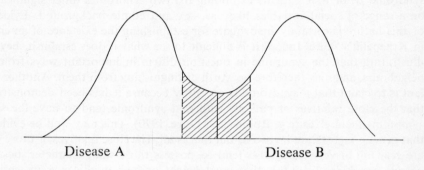

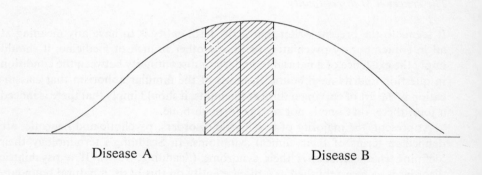

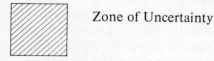  Zone of Uncertainty

*Figure 1.* Distributions of patients with and without a point of rarity.

This principle is fundamental to all classifications. It applies to butterflies and algae just as much as to diseases. As the bacteriologist Sneath (1957) observed in a thoughtful discussion of the principles underlying the classification of bacteria: 'We place the lines of division where the resultant groups will hold the greatest content of information. There are "points of rarity" in the distribution of features where individuals with certain combinations of features are rare, and since we are studying the world as it is we will place the divisions at the points of rarity. If there is no "point of rarity" it is useless to make a division.' Insistence on the presence of a 'point of rarity' is partly for the obvious reason that we are trying to put our boundaries where nature has hers, but it also has a strictly empirical justification. In practice there is bound to be some degree of error in identifying the exact position of each individual on the distribution, and hence for those who lie near the boundary, some doubt which side of it they lie. If the boundary is drawn at a point of rarity the proportion of the population affected in this way will be relatively small, whereas if the boundary is drawn at the peak of a distribution curve it will be unacceptably large (see Figure 1).

It must be emphasized that this distribution does not represent a single symptom or the score on any single rating scale. In practice, where clinical syndromes are concerned, it will generally be a complex dimension derived from all the different symptoms which serve to define the syndrome in question and its derivation may involve multivariate statistical techniques like discriminant function analysis (see chapter 8).

## The search for discontinuities

At present there is not a single functional psychiatric disorder which has been convincingly shown to be separated from other neighbouring syndromes by points of rarity, or where the relevant distribution curve has been shown to be bimodal. In spite of numerous casual claims to the contrary, we have not yet established the existence of any disease entities within our territory. As I have pointed out, in most cases where the claim has been made the substantiating evidence cited takes the form of a demonstration that the syndrome in question has a significantly different prognosis or response to treatment from other neighbouring syndromes, or is encountered in people with a significantly different age, sex or social class distribution. It should be clear from this discussion that evidence of this type is quite inadequate to establish a syndrome as an entity in the sense proposed here. Such evidence may serve to establish that the syndrome under consideration is a useful concept and worthy of further study, but that is all.

A few exceptions must be made to this generalization, however. Carney, Roth and Garside (1965) have claimed that there is a genuine boundary between what they call 'endogenous 'and 'neurotic' depressions. More recently, Gurney, Roth,

Garside, Kerr and Shapira (1972) have demonstrated a similar boundary between depressions as a whole and anxiety states, thus implying the existence of a second discontinuity between depressive neuroses and anxiety states. In each case, the nature of the evidence put forward, a bimodal distribution curve on a dimension derived by discriminant function analysis from an unselected population, is adequate in principle to establish the presence of at least one separate entity. However, neither study has yet been replicated by other workers, and attempts to do so for Carney's study have been unsuccessful (Kendell, 1969; Post, 1972). It is this lack of confirmation, rather than any inherent deficiencies in the evidence put forward, that leads the writer to conclude that, as yet, we have not established the existence of any functional disease entities.

### Continuity and discontinuity in organic disease

So far, this discussion has been confined to a consideration of diagnoses defined in terms of their clinical characteristics. At present most psychiatric diagnoses are defined in this way, but some are not and in other branches of medicine such diagnoses have dwindled to a small minority. For the majority, increasing knowledge of aetiology has moved their defining characteristic onto some other more fundamental plane. This may be an anatomical disturbance (as in mitral stenosis), a physiological disturbance (as in myasthenia gravis), a biochemical anomaly (as in phenylketonuria), an infective agent (as in tuberculosis), or a genetic or chromosomal anomaly (as in Down's syndrome). In principle at least, whichever of these levels its defining characteristic is drawn from an illness still may or may not be an entity. Whether it is depends on the same criterion as before, whether a discontinuity or natural boundary is involved. Down's syndrome is an entity because it is caused by, and defined by the presence of, a particular chromosomal anomaly which in any given individual can only be present or absent. (The phenomenon of mosaicism complicates this issue, but does not invalidate the principle.) Essential hypertension is not an entity, in spite of its undoubted genetic basis, because that basis is multifactorial, and therefore usually present only in partial form. Although the defining characteristic of a disease entity is frequently a qualitative deviation like an abnormal gene, which can only be present or absent, it need not be. The abnormality of thyroid metabolism responsible for thyrotoxicosis is essentially a quantitative deviation from normality which is capable of being present in varying extent. But in spite of the existence of some people with mild thyrotoxicosis, the illness is still an entity because in practice most people are either euthyroid or definitely thyrotoxic. Mild cases are relatively infrequent and so the distribution curve is bimodal (Crooks, Murray and Wayne, 1959). In essence therefore, the criterion whether a disease is or is not an entity remains the same regardless of the nature of its defining characteristic.

*The importance of the search for discontinuity.*

There are many reasons why it is important to establish whether or not the familiar syndromes of psychiatry, like schizophrenia and manic depressive illness, are genuine entities or not. Consider the consequences that would ensue if, for example, schizophrenia or some part of that syndrome proved to be an entity. Disagreements about which patients ought to be regarded as schizophrenics would be largely eliminated, because the point of rarity in the distribution curve demonstrating that it was an entity would ipso facto indicate where the boundary delineating schizophrenia from other syndromes should be. Furthermore, the argument between those advocating a dimensional classification and those favouring a typology would be resolved firmly in favour of the latter. However, the most important implication of such a demonstration would be the existence of another discontinuity further back in the causal chain. In order for the symptomatology of schizophrenia to be distinct, not merging insensibly into other syndromes, it would have to be dependent on the presence of some more fundamental qualitative anomaly, in the same way that the distinctive clinical presentation of Down's syndrome is dependent on the presence of an additional chromosome. The underlying anomaly need not necessarily be genetic. It could be physiological or even psychological, but it is almost impossible to visualize how a discontinuity could exist at a symptomatic level without being a reflection of a more fundamental discontinuity elsewhere.

Contemporary attempts to identify disease entities either at a clinical or a biochemical level are often scorned, particularly by behavioural scientists who see the attempt as evidence of the inability of psychiatrists to rid themselves of an outmoded 'medical model'. The attempt is still worthwhile in spite of being unfashionable. It is probably unlikely that any of the major syndromes of psychiatry will ever prove to be an entity in any strict sense, but if one did it would be a matter of unusual importance. For the reasons adumbrated above, it would almost certainly lead in time to major therapeutic innovations, and might well alter the whole trend of current thinking about the nature of mental illness, and the direction and scope of future research. With issues of such magnitude at stake it is well worthwhile for a few research teams to risk incurring the scepticism of their colleagues and the risk of eventual disappointment.

# 6 International Differences in Diagnostic Criteria

During the last two decades it has become apparent that there are a number of important, in some cases gross, differences in the diagnostic criteria used in different parts of the world, and even between different centres in a single country. Although the demonstration of these differences was initially greeted with pained surprise, their existence is an almost inevitable consequence of the means by which psychiatrists have traditionally assigned diagnoses to their patients.

*How and why differences arise*

Consider how trainee psychiatrists learn which diagnoses to apply to their patients. They begin by learning the typical clinical features of different diagnostic categories from lectures and textbooks. They learn that schizophrenia is characterized by delusions of control, thought disorder, blunting of affect and a downhill course; that involutional melancholia is characterized by severe agitation, bizarre hypochondriacal or nihilistic delusions and the absence of earlier episodes of depression, and so on. They quickly come to realize, however, that this knowledge is of only limited use because the majority of the patients they encounter do not possess these neat clusters of symptoms. They have some of them, certainly, but others are missing, and often they have additional symptoms which ought to belong to some other category. As a result, the student is forced to learn how to assign diagnoses largely by personal example. He sees which sorts of patients his teachers regard as schizophrenics, and copies them. Moreover, he has to use this same modelling process to find out which patients to label as thought disordered, rather than simply as wooly-minded, and which to label as retarded, rather than merely as ponderous or lazy. In short, although trainees are provided with typical examples of the sorts of behaviour to which symptom concepts like thought disorder and higher level diagnostic concepts like schizophrenia are applicable, they are not given clear definitions or rules

70

of application for either, nor is the relationship between the two specified clearly.

As a result, diagnostic concepts are not securely anchored. They are at the mercy of the personal views and idiosyncracies of influential teachers, of therapeutic fashions and innovations, of changing assumptions about aetiology, and many other less tangible influences to boot. If a new and seemingly effective treatment is introduced, those diagnostic categories to which it is applicable tend to expand at the expense of others to which it is not. If a diagnosis acquires pejorative connotations or a reputation for being untreatable, its sphere of application tends to shrink, except perhaps in patients with whom the diagnostician is out of sympathy. If ideas about the aetiology of a diagnostic category change, the sorts of patients to whom that diagnosis is applied also tend to change in such a way as to maximize the plausibility of the new theory. Because of our lack of firm criteria, such changes are taking place all the time, and occurring at different speeds and to differing extents in different centres. So whenever two centres are sufficiently remote from one another for communication to be difficult and interchange of staff infrequent differences in diagnostic criteria between the two are likely to develop. As national boundaries and language differences inevitably hinder free communication and the diffusion of ideas, international differences in diagnostic criteria are almost inevitable, and will remain so until we change our ways.

ANGLO-AMERICAN DIFFERENCES

The most well known and extensively studied international differences are those between Britain and the United States. It has long been known that there are considerable differences between the diagnostic statistics generated by the mental hospitals of these two countries. These were commented on many years ago by Slater (1935), and later by Lewis (1946), but were first examined systematically by Kramer (1961). Kramer calculated first admission rates for various diagnostic categories from the data published by the Ministry of Health for England and Wales, compared these with the corresponding rates for public and private hospitals in the United States, and found several striking differences between the two. The first admission rate for schizophrenia was half as high again in the United States as in England and Wales and the first admission rate for cerebral arteriosclerosis ten times as high. For manic depressive illness, on the other hand, the rate was nine times higher in England and Wales that in the United States, and for some age groups the difference was as high as twentyfold.

In principle, there are three possible explanations for such differences. They might be due to genuine differences in the prevalence of different types of mental illness in the two countries. Alternatively they might be due, in the absence of differences in prevalence, to different sorts of patients gaining admission to hospital as a result of differences in referral or admission practices. Or they might be due to differences in diagnostic criteria, that is to American and British psychiatrists attaching different diagnostic labels to patients with identical symptoms. In fact it has now been established that, in this instance, differences in diagnostic criteria are largely responsible.

## The Diagnostic Project studies

Some 10 years ago an Anglo-American research team, known as the US/UK Diagnostic Project, was created in order to investigate the differences which Kramer had drawn attention to. Their first studies were designed to find out how much of the diagnostic differences between the two countries would disappear if series of patients entering hospital in each were examined and diagnosed by identical means. Two hundred and fifty consecutive admissions between the ages of 20 and 59 were studied at a single hospital in each country, Netherne Hospital south of London, and the Brooklyn State Hospital in New York City.

TABLE 1 Hospital and 'Project' diagnoses of samples of patients admitted to public mental hospitals in New York and London.

| Diagnosis | Hospital Diagnoses | | | | 'Project' Diagnoses | | | |
|---|---|---|---|---|---|---|---|---|
| | New York patients | | London patients | | New York patients | | London patients | |
| | No. | % | No. | % | No. | % | No. | % |
| Schizophrenia | 118 | 61.5 | 59 | 33.9** | 56 | 29.2 | 61 | 35.1 |
| Depressive psychoses | 9 | 4.7 | 42 | 24.1** | 38 | 19.8 | 40 | 23.0 |
| Mania | 1 | 0.5 | 12 | 6.9** | 11 | 5.7 | 11 | 6.3 |
| Depressive neuroses | 3 | 1.6 | 14 | 8.0** | 13 | 6.8 | 25 | 14.4* |
| Other neuroses | 5 | 2.6 | 10 | 5.7 | 3 | 1.6 | 7 | 4.0 |
| Personality disorders | 2 | 1.0 | 8 | 4.6* | 8 | 4.2 | 5 | 2.9 |
| Alcoholic disorders | 38 | 19.8 | 6 | 3.4** | 44 | 22.9 | 8 | 4.6** |
| Drug dependence | 0 | — | 1 | 0.6 | 6 | 3.1 | 1 | 0.6 |
| Organic psychoses | 10 | 5.2 | 3 | 1.7 | 5 | 2.6 | 6 | 3.4 |
| Other diagnoses | 6 | 3.1 | 19 | 10.9** | 8 | 4.2 | 10 | 5.7 |

\*\**difference significant at the 1 per cent level*
\* *difference significant at the 5 per cent level*

Information was obtained, by structured interviewing methods, from the patients and their relatives and a diagnosis assigned to each patient on this basis, using the nomenclature of the 8th edition of the *International Classification* and the British glossary to this (General Register Office, 1968). The 'project diagnoses' obtained in this way were then compared with the diagnoses given independently to the same patients by the hospital staff. Although the two sets of hospital diagnoses were very different from one another, and reflected the familiar differences between the national statistics of the two countries, the differences between the two sets of project diagnoses were much more modest. Indeed, the only significant difference was a higher proportion of patients with depressive illnesses in the English series (Cooper, Kendell, Gurland, Sharpe, Copeland and Simon, 1972).

Subsequently the same authors carried out a similar comparison between a sample of 192 patients drawn from the nine state hospitals supplying New York City and an analogous sample of 174 patients drawn from nine of the eighteen area mental hospitals supplying Greater London. The results of this inter-city comparison, shown in Table 1, were essentially the same as those of the original single hospital comparison. There were significant differences between the two sets of hospital diagnoses for almost every major diagnostic category, but when these were replaced by the uniform criteria of the 'project diagnoses' most of these differences disappeared. Alcoholic disorders remained significantly commoner in the New York patients, and depressive neuroses in the London patients, but the large differences between the proportions of patients given hospital diagnoses of schizophrenia, depressive psychosis and mania were all greatly reduced and ceased to be significant.

If one assumes that the project diagnoses in these two studies were made to identical criteria in both countries, and great care was taken to ensure this by an exchange of interviewers between London and New York and numerous statistical checks on consistency, it follows that there must be substantial differences between the diagnostic criteria used by London psychiatrists and New York psychiatrists. With the single exception of alcoholism every major diagnostic category seems to be involved, though it is likely that several of these differences are secondary to the gross disparity in use of the term schizophrenia. Over 60 per cent of the New York patients received hospital diagnoses of schizophrenia, compared with less than 30 per cent of the London sample. Indeed, if alcoholics and patients with organic psychoses are excluded, only 18 per cent of the New York patients (26 out of 144) received any other diagnosis. To look at the matter the other way round, the four diagnoses of depressive psychosis, mania, neurosis and personality disorder were all used fairly frequently by the London hospital staff, and between them account for 49 per cent of their hospital diagnoses. None of the four was used at all frequently by the New York hospital staff, and between them they account for only 10 per cent of their diagnoses. The all-inclusive nature of New York psychiatrists' concept of schizophrenia is vividly illustrated by the fact that over 60 per cent of the patients with project diagnoses of depressive psychosis, neurosis or personality disorder all had hospital diagnoses of schizophrenia, and for mania the figure was over 90 per cent.

6

*Anglo-American videotape comparisons*

A more direct way of comparing the diagnostic criteria of two groups of psychiatrists is to show films or videotapes of diagnostic interviews to both and compare the diagnoses they make. Several such comparisons have been carried out between audiences of American and British psychiatrists with results that broadly confirm those of these hospital admission comparisons. (See Sandifer, Hordern, Timbury and Green, 1968; Katz, Cole and Lowery, 1969; Kendell, Cooper, Gourlay, Copeland, Sharpe and Gurland, 1971.) In the third of these studies, videotaped interviews of eight patients (five English and three American) were shown to audiences of up to 200 experienced psychiatrists on both sides of the Atlantic. Some of the patients were picked as typical cases and others deliberately chosen in the expectation that they might give rise to diagnostic disagreement. For the three patients whose symptoms were similar to those of classical textbook descriptions there was substantial agreement between American and British psychiatrists, at least for the major category of illness involved. For three other patients with both schizophrenic and affective symptoms the majority of both American and British raters diagnosed schizophrenia, but for all three a substantial minority of British raters preferred to diagnose an affective psychosis. For the last two patients there was serious disagreement, most British raters diagnosing either a personality disorder or a neurotic illness, and the majority of the Americans again diagnosing schizophrenia.

The full distribution of diagnoses given to one of these patients is shown in Table 2. The disagreement could hardly be more flagrant, particularly as over 80 per cent of both audiences indicated that they were confident in their respective diagnoses. The patient concerned was a 30-year-old bachelor from Brooklyn who had never had frank psychotic symptoms but had been in hospital briefly several times, had no close friends, and had rarely held a steady job. In the interview he described having once had a hysterical paralysis of his arm, and gave a vivid account of the fluctuations in his mood and morale and of his willingness to abuse alcohol or drugs whenever opportunity arose. Most British raters regarded him as having a hysterical personality disorder, whereas the Americans regarded him as a schizophrenic, many commenting that his symptoms were typical of pseudoneurotic schizophrenia. A similar disparity between the diagnoses of American and British audiences was reported by Katz for his aspiring actress patient (Katz, Cole and Lowery, 1969).

The Diagnostic Project group summarized these Anglo-American differences in the form of a Venn diagram, reproduced in Figure 2, which shows the American concept of schizophrenia embracing substantial parts of what British psychiatrists would regard as depressive illness, neurotic illness or personality disorder and most of what they would regard as mania. This frightening disparity needs qualifying somewhat in the light of subsequent events and more recent findings. Most of the Anglo-American comparisons described above were primarily comparisons between London and New York. It has now become clear that there are substantial differences in diagnostic criteria between different centres in the United States and that the New York concept of schizophrenia is unusually comprehensive even by North American standards. Sharpe and his colleagues carried out a videotape study involving several different training centres in the United States and Canada and found that psychiatrists in California and Illinois were less prone to diagnose schizophrenia than their colleagues on the eastern seaboard, though still having a much wider concept than the British, and Sandifer's earlier work had suggested previously that the differences between North Carolina and Britain were relatively modest. So to some extent this diagram gives too alarming a picture of the overall national difference. It is also likely that, if these studies were to be repeated now, American psychiatrists would be found much readier to diagnose mania than they were in the 1960's. Certainly the introduction of lithium as a specific treatment for mania towards the end of that decade produced a dramatic resurgence of interest in the diagnosis. Indeed several authors have commented on the 'epidemic' of mania that appeared to sweep through the eastern United States at that time.

TABLE 2 Diagnoses made by American and British psychiatrists after seeing the same video-taped diagnostic interview.

| Diagnosis | American Psychiatrists (N = 133) | British Psychiatrists (N = 194) |
|---|---|---|
| *Schizophrenia* | 92 (69%) | 4 (2%) |
| Simple | 0 | 1 |
| Catatonic | 1 | 0 |
| Paranoid | 27 | 1 |
| Latent | 8 | 0 |
| Residual | 3 | 0 |
| Schizo-affective | 33 | 1 |
| Unspecified | 20 | 1 |
| *Personality disorder* | 10 (8%) | 146 (75%) |
| Paranoid | 1 | 2 |
| Affective (cyclothymic) | 1 | 8 |
| Explosive | 0 | 2 |
| Hysterical | 4 | 105 |
| Asthenic | 0 | 2 |
| Antisocial | 1 | 8 |
| Unspecified | 3 | 19 |
| *Affective psychosis* | 10 (8%) | 7 (4%) |
| *Neurosis* | 19 (14%) | 37 (19%) |
| *Alcoholism or drug dependence* | 2 | 0 |

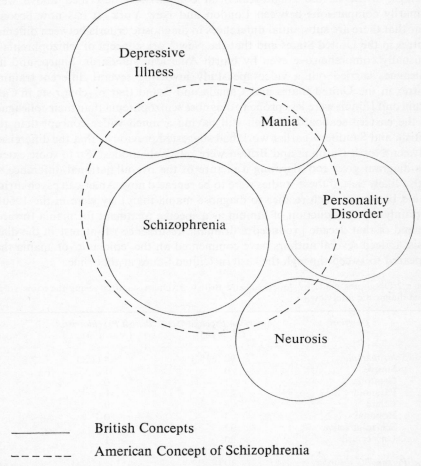

_____  British Concepts

_ _ _ _ _  American Concept of Schizophrenia

*Figure* 2. The contrast between American and British concepts of schizophrenia (US/UK Diagnostic project, 1971).

OTHER INTERNATIONAL DIFFERENCES

Other international differences are less well documented but enough work has been done to make the main outlines of the situation reasonably clear. Overall and a series of European collaborators compared the diagnostic stereotypes of American, French, German, Italian and Czechoslovakian psychiatrists. They did so by asking groups of experienced psychiatrists in each of these countries to invent Brief Psychiatric Rating Scale, (i.e. mental state), ratings for hypothetical typical patients from each of the different categories of psychosis they recognized, and then comparing these profiles with one another, first within and then between the different countries involved. Their results indicated that the broad concepts of schizophrenia, mania and depression used in these five countries were all very similar. But there were several differences in the sub-categories of schizophrenia and depression that were recognized, in the symptomatology attributed to each, and also in the range of other paranoid or hallucinatory psychoses recognized (Pichot, Bailly and Overall, 1966; Engelsmann, Vinar, Pichot, Hippius, Giberti, Rossi and Overall, 1970).

While these stereotype comparisons were in progress, Rawnsley (1967) compared the diagnoses attributed to a series of thirty patients by groups of psychiatrists from five different countries – 260 in the USA, 205 in the UK, twenty eight in Norway, eighteen in Sweden and thirty in Denmark. The patients were picked at random from admissions to a British area mental hospital and the study was based entirely on 400 word case summaries in English. A clear trend emerged for American psychiatrists to diagnose schizophrenia where European psychiatrists diagnosed depression, obsessional disorder or paranoid psychosis, and for Scandinavian psychiatrists to diagnose psychogenic psychosis where the British and the Americans tended to diagnose neurotic illness. In a later WHO study, designed to shed some light on the Scandinavian concept of psychogenic psychosis, patients diagnosed as having reactive or psychogenic psychoses by Norwegian and Danish psychiatrists were often regarded as schizophrenics or manic depressives by others; and it was clear that use of the term reactive psychosis was variable even within the three Scandinavian countries (Astrup and Ødegaard, 1970).

Although there is no particular reason to doubt the results of any of these studies their limitations must not be overlooked. Overall's findings must be treated with caution in view of Sandifer's demonstration that hypothetical stereotype ratings are an unreliable guide to the way diagnoses are used in practice (Hordern, Sandifer, Green and Timbury, 1968). Rawnsley's study almost certainly provides an underestimate of the severity of diagnostic variation, because it was based entirely on written summaries which eliminate what may well be the most important source of variation, the observer's own perception of psychopathology. It was probably for this reason that an early WHO study (Shepherd, Brooke, Cooper and Lin, 1968) failed to elicit worse disagreement within a group of psychiatrists from eight different countries than within a group of English psychiatrists.

## Differences within Europe

We have some information about diagnostic criteria on the continent of Europe from a videotape comparison organized by Kendell, Pichot and von Cranach

(1974). Videotape recordings were made of brief diagnostic interviews, lasting exactly 5 minutes each, with an unselected series of twenty seven patients newly admitted to a psychiatric hospital in London. These videotapes were then shown to groups of experienced psychiatrists in London, Paris and Munich who were required to make a diagnosis and a number of other ratings for each. All the members of the French and German audiences spoke fairly fluent English, and were also provided with verbatim transcripts of the interviews in an attempt to compensate for the greater difficulty they inevitably experienced in understanding and evaluating the dialogue between patient and interviewer. The results of this study indicated that the three groups all had much the same global concepts of schizophrenia and neurotic illness, and probably of personality disorder and alcoholism also. But they differed markedly in the realm of affective illness. The broadest concepts of both psychotic and neurotic depression, and also of mania, were all held by the English audience and the narrowest by the French. The cardinal difference between the three appeared to be manic depressive illness, which accounted for 23 per cent of all diagnoses made by the London raters, compared with 14 per cent for Munich and a mere 5 per cent for Paris. A variety of different labels were given by the French psychiatrists to the patients the English regarded an manic depressives, including involutional melancholia, alcoholism and schizophrenia. Overall, the ratings of the English and German audiences were much closer to one another than either was to the French. Indeed, comparable differences might well have been obtained between different centres in the same country. To what extent these results are indicative of national differences depends on how typical the dozen psychiatrists constituting each of the three audiences were of their respective countries. There is some evidence that the diagnostic criteria used in London do not differ appreciably from those used elsewhere in the British Isles (Copeland, Cooper, Kendell and Gourlay, 1971) but we have no factual information at present about the extent of variation from centre to centre within France and Germany.

*Translation problems*

All the studies mentioned so far, apart from Overall's stereotype comparisons, were restricted either to English-speaking countries, or to English speaking psychiatrists working elsewhere. The reason for this is not hard to find. As psychiatric diagnoses are largely based on what patients say, rather than on other aspects of their behaviour, psychiatrists can only be asked to diagnose patients who were interviewed in a language they speak reasonably fluently themselves. It is, of course, perfectly possible to translate case histories into other languages, or to translate structured interviews or rating scales. It would even be possible to dub films or videotapes of diagnostic interviews in other languages as is done routinely with commercial films. But translation holds many unsuspected pitfalls even when checked by back translation and carried out by people thoroughly familiar with both languages and with psychiatry.

Sartorius describes several of these in his account of the linguistic problems encountered in the *International Pilot Study of Schizophrenia* (WHO, 1973a). A vivid example quoted by Lehmann (1971) serves to illustrate the scale of the problem. The question 'How is your mind working?' in Spitzer's Present Status Schedule (PSS) was translated into French as 'Comment votre cerveau, votre esprit, fonctionne-t-il?' This PSS item qualifies for a positive rating if the patient in his reply 'mentions his thinking is impaired, or that he keeps losing his train of thought, or that he can't concentrate'. In a population of English speaking Canadians 60 per cent of depressives but only 5 per cent of schizophrenics gave replies meriting a positive rating, but in a comparable population of French speaking Canadians there was a dramatic reversal of the ratio with 40 per cent of schizophrenics and only 15 per cent of depressives producing positive ratings. Presumably these apparently analogous questions have important differences in meaning to English and French Canadian patients that were not apparent to the bilingual psychiatrists responsible for the translation. An even worse problem is that a word or phrase with strong diagnostic implications in one language may not exist in another, or two feeling or mood states with different diagnostic connotations in one language may be embraced by a single term in another. For example, some languages, like the Yoruba tongue of Western Nigeria, have no word for depression, and in Chinese no distinction is made between worry and anxiety. A more familiar problem is the German word angst which has no counterpart in English and has to be rendered inadequately as anxiety, and einsam which carries with it heroic undertones that are entirely lacking in the English word loneliness.

Unfortunately, these problems have to be accepted if we wish to compare diagnostic criteria in countries with different languages. In recent years widely used structured English language interviews like the Present State Examination (PSE) and the Psychiatric Status Schedule have been translated into several other languages. Once this has been done, and bearing in mind the hazards involved, diagnostic criteria in countries with different languages can be compared indirectly by comparing the relationships between ratings and diagnoses in each.

*The International Pilot Study of Schizophrenia*

Although this was not its main purpose, the *International Pilot Study of Schizophrenia* provides invaluable information about diagnostic criteria in just this way. Indeed, it provides the only reliable information we possess about diagnostic criteria outside North America and Western Europe. Analysis of the relationship between PSE ratings and diagnoses by means of the computer program Catego (see chapter 11) showed that in seven of the nine regional centres involved in the project – in London, Prague, Aarhus in Denmark, Ibadan in Nigeria, Agra in India, Cali in Colombia and Taipeh in Formosa – the local psychiatrists all had substantially the same concept of schizophrenia. However, in the other two, Moscow and Washington, a considerably broader concept prevailed. The American concept of schizophrenia has already been discussed. The Russian concept of this illness embraces three sub-types, periodic, sluggish and shift-like schizophrenia, which are not recognized elsewhere. In general, Russian psychiatrists appear to be influenced more by the course of the illness and less by its actual symptomatology than other European psychiatrists, a fact which has some bearing on recent political controversies.

It was suggested at the beginning of this chapter that disparities in diagnostic criteria arise on a basis of inadequate communication, and that for this reason they should tend to be most obvious between centres isolated from one another by language or distance, and greater between one country and another than between different centres in the same country. In general this appears to be so, though there are some notable exceptions, for example the much greater differences between London and New York than between London and Munich.

## Differences within the British Isles

Within the relatively compact and homogenous area of the British Isles there is little evidence of significant variation from one centre to another. Copeland, Cooper, Kendell and Gourlay (1971) showed videotapes of diagnostic interviews with three different patients to audiences of experienced psychiatrists in seven different cities – London, Birmingham, Manchester, Edinburgh, Glasgow, Belfast and Dublin. For two of the three patients no significant diagnostic differences emerged, regardless of whether the two hundred psychiatrists involved were grouped by the region in which they were currently working or by the centre at which they had originally trained. And for the third patient, a woman with both schizophrenic and affective symptoms, only one significant difference emerged. Psychiatrists who had originally been trained in Glasgow were relatively more disposed than their colleagues elsewhere to diagnose an affective psychosis rather than schizophrenia.

## Differences within North America

As might have been predicted from the greater distances involved, larger differences exist between one centre and another in North America. Sharpe and his colleagues showed videotapes of patients who had previously been found to elicit diagnostic disagreements between psychiatrists in New York and in the British Isles to audiences in several different Canadian and American centres. Although the broad New York concept of schizophrenia extended to other neighbouring cities it did not extend to Illinois or California, and Sandifer had shown previously that it did not extend to North Carolina. In general terms, there seems to be a gradient across the United States from east to west, though even in California the prevailing concept of schizophrenia is considerably broader than in Britain. The only American centres where this does not appear to be so are St. Louis and Iowa where the criteria currently used to diagnose both schizophrenia and manic depressive illness are very similar to those used in England or Germany. Canadian criteria were generally found to be intermediate between those of the British and the Americans, though tending to be closer to the latter and to vary from place to place. In Toronto, for example, the prevailing criteria were relatively 'English' in character. In general, the criteria adopted in the Canadian centres that were visited seemed to reflect the relative numbers of American and English trained psychiatrists on the University faculty. (Sharpe, Gurland, Fleiss, Kendell, Cooper and Copeland, 1974).

THE CAUSE OF THE DIFFERENCES

For the most part it is still unclear which aspects of the diagnostic process are involved in the various differences that have been described, or indeed how they arose historically, but some information is available where the Anglo-American differences are concerned and may be of wider relevance. At least in this instance, differences in diagnostic stereotypes do not seem to be important because, despite using several key terms like schizophrenia and manic depressive illness in very different ways, American and British psychiatrists appear to agree closely on the characteristic symptoms of these conditions. Hordern, Sandifer, Green and Timbury (1968) asked small groups of psychiatrists in North Carolina, London and Glasgow to list in order of importance the typical symptoms of twenty of the most commonly used diagnostic categories. They found inter–group differences to be small and no greater than intra–group differences, in spite of the fact that they had previously demonstrated several inter–group differences in actual usage amongst these same psychiatrists. A similar finding emerged from the London/Paris/Munich comparison described above. Although the English and French psychiatrists involved in that study used diagnoses like depression and mania quite differently, they rated the same features as being of diagnostic importance in these conditions.

Apart from differences in diagnostic stereotypes there are, in principle, three other possible explanations for the observed discrepancies. First, the apparent similarity between the stereotypes held by different schools of psychiatry may be illusory because the technical terms used to define the diagnoses in question may themselves hold different meanings for them. American and British psychiatrists may agree, for example, that schizophrenia is characterized by thought disorder and flattening of affect, but mean different things by flattening of affect and thought disorder. Secondly, disagreement may occur because one group insists on a much closer correspondence than the other between the symptoms of the patient and those of the stereotype before being prepared to accept that diagnosis as established. Thirdly, the two may actually perceive, or recognize, different abnormalities in spite of observing the same behavioural phenomena. At least where the Anglo-American differences are concerned, it seems likely that there are significant differences at each of these levels and that the observed differences in usage are the cumulative product of all three.

The videotape comparisons described previously provide many examples of what appear to be perceptual differences between American and British raters. Both Katz *et al.* (1969) and Kendell *et al.* (1971) found significant differences between the ratings of their American and British audiences on Lorr's In-Patient Multidimensional Psychiatric Scale (Lorr and Klett, 1967), although this instrument avoids all technical terms and its ratings purport to be straightforward, linear measures of deviation from normality. It has, in fact, been an invariable finding that American psychiatrists rate higher on this scale on both American and English patients in all areas of psychopathology, but particularly so in those with strong schizophrenic connotations. When ratings involving technical terms are compared, however, much larger differences are liable to be obtained. For instance, the subject of one of the videotaped interviews used by the Diagnostic Project team, was rated by 67 per cent of a group of 133 American psychiatrists as having delusions, by 63 per cent as having passivity feelings, and by 58 per cent as showing thought disorder. The corresponding percentages for an audience of 194 British psychiatrists were 12 per cent for delusions, 8 per cent for passivity feelings, and 5 per cent for thought disorder. The fact that these discrepancies are so much worse than those between the corresponding IMPS ratings strongly suggests that an important conceptual element is present on top of the perceptual difference. It suggests, in other words, that the two groups mean different things by thought disorder and passivity feelings as well as perceiving or recognizing rather different deviations from normal behaviour in the first place.

*'Ragbag' categories*

Although there is little evidence bearing directly on the issue, it seems likely that there are also important differences between American and British psychiatrists in the degree of similarity between the patient's symptoms and those of the diagnostic stereotype which the two require to establish particular diagnoses, and that this makes an important contribution to the observed differences in usage. Because many patients do not fit neatly into well-defined diagnostic categories every classification has to have, in practice if not in theory, at least one category which is only loosely defined and can act as a 'ragbag' for patients who do not fit in elsewhere. It was the impression of the Diagnostic Project team that patients with nondescript symptoms tended to be diagnosed as schizophrenics by New York psychiatrists at least in part because other diagnoses like manic depressive illness were ruled out by the very close correspondence required between the patient's symptoms and those of this stereotype before a diagnosis of manic depressive illness could be made. In London, on the other hand, the situation tended to be the other way about. Close agreement between the patient's symptoms and those of the stereotype was often insisted upon for a diagnosis of schizophrenia, but much greater latitude was allowed for diagnoses of depressive illness, affective psychosis or personality disorder. If one is prepared to take seriously the dictum that 'even a trace of schizophrenia is schizophrenia' it is very easy to use schizophrenia as a ragbag diagnosis; and mood disturbances are so ubiquitous that there is little difficulty in doing the same for affective disorders.

*Bronchitis v. emphysema*

Serious differences in diagnostic criteria are not a problem only for psychiatry. It is not so long since chest physicians discovered that the apparent predominance of chronic bronchitis in England and of emphysema in North America was largely due to the fact that the constellation of symptoms and pulmonary deficits known as chronic bronchitis in London was diagnosed as emphysema in Chicago (Fletcher, Jones, Burrows and Niden, 1964). But the situation is more serious in psychiatry than in other branches of medicine because most psychiatric diagnoses are still defined by their syndromes, and constellations of symptoms are much harder to convert into unambiguous definitions than biochemical or histological abnormalities.

*Impairment of communication*

The importance of the variations in diagnostic criteria that have been described here lies in the grave effects they are liable to have on communication. Diagnoses are the most important of all psychiatry's technical terms because they are the means by which the subject matter of most psychiatric research is identified. They are the means used by both clinicians and research workers to convey to others the essential attributes of the patients they are talking or writing about. If different people use these labels in different ways they will at best fail to communicate accurately, and may well actively mislead one another. A single example will serve to illustrate the point. The fact that American and British psychiatrists mean different things by schizophrenia, and probably have done for over thirty years, means that throughout this time each has been both misunderstanding and misleading the other. The fact that both are now aware of the differences reduces the confusion somewhat, but the two still lack the common language they must have if transatlantic communication is ever to be straightforward. Awareness of the differences that previously went unrecognized also necessitates an extensive reappraisal by British psychiatrists of much American research, and vice versa. The significance to British psychiatrists of, for example, Lidz's well known studies of the families of schizophrenics (Lidz, Fleck and Cornelison, 1965), and the aetiological theories derived from these, cannot fail to be affected by the suspicion that they themselves would not have regarded most of the patients on whom this work was based as schizophrenics in the first place. Conversely, American psychiatrists may well need to revise their assessment of several British studies of depressive illness now that they realize that many of the patients involved were probably not suffering from depression in the sense in which they understand that term.

In future it should be harder for the diagnostic criteria used in different countries to diverge from one another than it has been in the past. Awareness of existing differences and the grave difficulties they pose is itself some protection. And the increasing scope and ease of international travel and communication make it much harder for individual countries or training centres to remain in isolation from outside influences. Clinicians and research workers both attend conferences abroad, work in other countries for substantial periods and read foreign journals far more often than they did a generation or even a decade ago.

*The elimination of differences*

To eliminate existing differences is a much harder problem. If psychiatrists detected the same abnormalities in patients to whom they attributed different diagnoses the problem would be relatively simple. Patients could be identified by their symptoms instead of by diagnoses, and different schools of psychiatry might even be persuaded to agree on common definitions for their diagnoses. But, as we have seen, disagreements over which symptoms the patient exhibits are sometimes just as flagrant as disagreements over diagnosis. Whether clinicians make different diagnoses because they detect different symptoms, or detect different symptoms because they have already recognized a familiar illness, is an important and intriguing issue. Either way, the fact that perceptual differences are involved as well as purely conceptual ones makes it hard for someone who has been trained in one frame of reference to change to another. The provision of a carefully worded operational definition for each diagnostic category, and also for key symptoms like thought disorder, would make things much easier, but not reduce the extent of the upheaval. We would all be happy for other people to change into step with ourselves, but probably few of us are prepared to make the considerable effort involved in changing our own established habits in order to conform with them. And of course we have no firm criteria for deciding whether A ought to change in order to conform with B, or whether B ought to do so in order to conform with A. We may argue that one concept of schizophrenia is more useful than another, or closer to Bleuler's original concept, but until our diagnoses are defined at some more fundamental level than their clinical syndromes, we cannot maintain that one concept is right and others wrong.* In short, no one is likely to abandon his habitual diagnostic behaviour in favour of someone else's unless he is given a compelling reason for doing so, and no such reason exists, beyond the need for uniformity. For this reason, it is likely that major changes in existing diagnostic concepts will only occur after, and as a consequence of, therapeutic innovations or biochemical or physiological discoveries. The changes that have recently taken place in the American concept of mania illustrate this quite well. At one time, the diagnosis of mania was made much less often in the eastern United States than it was in Europe, Indeed in New York it was made so rarely that it was in some danger of becoming extinct. However, in the course of a few years the situation changed markedly, not because American psychiatrists suddenly realized that their concept of mania was idiosyncratic, but because they came to realize that lithium salts were an effective treatment for mania, and also that there was real hope of elucidation the chemical basis of the cyclical mood change in manic depressive illness, and so had strong motives to find manic patients to treat and study.

For the forseeable future, therefore, it is unrealistic to expect international differences in diagnostic criteria to fade away. The best we can hope for is that further important discrepancies will not develop, and that the ill effects of existing differences will be reduced by recognition of their existence. Their elimination will have to be a long term process, depending partly on the development and slowly increasing acceptance of an international nomenclature equipped with adequate operational definitions, and partly on the more potent effects of therapeutic and aetiological advances as and when these occur.

* This does not mean that it is impossible to produce rational criteria for preferring one concept to another. Shields and Gottesman (1973), for instance, have argued that an appropriate criterion for diseases with an established genetic basis like schizophrenia might be to choose whichever concept gave the highest MZ/DZ concordance ratio in twin populations. The preliminary data they present suggests, in fact, that the highest concordance ratio for schizophrenia is provided by very strict diagnostic criteria. Other equally rational, but none the less arbitrary, criteria could easily be invented, based on prognosis or therapeutic response.

# 7 The International Classification

If any man were bold enough to write a history of psychiatric classifications he would find when he had completed his task that in the process he had written a history of psychiatry as well. For the range and varieties of mental illness recognized in a classification, their names and their relationships with one another, reflect very accurately the assumptions and knowledge of its authors, their ideas about the nature of insanity and their familiarity with, or ignorance of, its manifestations. Karl Menninger has collected together many of the surviving classifications of the past 3000 years as a fascinating appendix to his book, the *Vital Balance* (Menninger, 1963). He starts with the classifications of Hippocrates, Plato and Celsus in the ancient world and slowly progresses to Galen, Avicenna, Robert Burton and Boissier de Sauvages, and finally ends with some hearty criticisms of the 1951 classification of the American Psychiatric Association. Some illnesses, like mania and melancholia, appear in almost every classification from Hippocrates onwards, changing their content and meaning insidiously from century to century. Others, like the Scythian disease of Hippocrates and the neophrenias of Kahlbaum, make one brief appearance and then vanish. Menninger professes to see in this long pageant a steady increase in complexity followed by a more healthy trend towards simplicity, and culminating in his own unitary concept of mental illness. It is certainly true that no other classifications before or since have matched the complexity, or the absurdity, of the classifications of Boissier de Sauvages and Cullen in the 18th century. But apart from this brief Byzantine episode, there has always been a fluctuating to and fro relationship between simplicity and complexity, complicated by the fact that many classifications are tiered, and so capable of appearing simple at one level and complex at another. In fact, in so far as there is an underlying trend, it is probably towards increasing complexity rather than simplicity, if only because our concept of mental illness has broadened steadily, particularly in the last hundred years, and the range of phenomena involved increased correspondingly. Before this century most classifications were really classifications of insanity as this was the only type of mental abnormality recognized as illness. Even the classification put forward by Kraepelin in the famous 6th (1899) edition of his *Lehrbuch* lumps all non-psychotic states together into three ill-defined groups at the end, called general neuroses (embracing both epilepsy and hysteria), psychopathic conditions (neurasthenia, homosexuality, etc.) and developmental inhibitions (imbecility and idiocy).

Before the closing years of the 18th century, most classifications of insanity were based on a very imperfect acquaintance with the actual phenomena of mental illness. They were produced by eminent physicians like Galen and Jean Fernel who were classifying insanity more or less incidentally in the course of elaborating a general classification of disease, or by philosophers like Plato and Kant. Some, like Thomas Willis, were well acquainted with the ways of lunatics but few were in any real sense specialists in the treatment of insanity and none had any close familiarity with the course of mental illness. But as cities began to grow in size and become industrialized, the social problems posed by the insane rapidly became more obtrusive. One by one cities throughout Europe were forced to build large asylums to house their lunatics, and appoint physicians to care for them. This new breed, men like Pinel and Esquirol, were not only more familiar with the phenomena of insanity than their predecessors, but were also for the first time able to observe the lifetime course of their charges' illnesses. From this time on, events moved swiftly and the pace quickened further with the establishment of university departments of psychiatry and neurology in several German cities in the latter half of the nineteenth century.

## The 19th century

For a long time confusion reigned. Every self-respecting alienist, and certainly every professor, had his own classification, some based on differences in behaviour, others on presumed differences in aetiology, often of the most fanciful kinds, others on differences in psychology, some on a combination of all three. As Zilboorg (1941) observed, 'to produce a well-ordered classification almost seemed to have become the unspoken ambition of every psychiatrist of industry and promise'. It soon became apparent that this multiplicity of classifications, with the same terms often having different meanings in different typologies, rendered communication between one hospital and another almost impossible, and with this came recognition of the need for a single classification acceptable to everyone. At the Congress of Mental Medicine held at Antwerp in 1885 a commission was appointed, under the chairmanship of M. Morel, to consider existing classifications and derive from them a single typology 'which the various associations of alienists could unite in adopting'. Four years later the International Congress of Mental Science in Paris duly adopted the classification recommended by this commission, but, as Hack Tuke subsequently remarked, 'it has yet to be seen whether asylum physicians will adopt it in their tables'

(Tuke, 1892). In fact Tuke's pessimism soon proved to be justified but, as the forerunner of our present international classification, the commission's typology deserves recording despite its early demise. It consisted of eleven categories, including all those 'upon which the majority (of the commission's members) was unanimous' and omitting those 'upon which opinion was divided' yet aspiring nonetheless to embrace all 'the principal forms of madness'. Tuke (1890) listed it thus:

### The International Classification of 1889.

1. Mania (comprising acute delirious mania)
2. Melancholia
3. Periodical insanity (folie à double forme)
4. Progressive systematic insanity
5. Dementia
6. Organic and senile dementia
7. General paralysis
8. Insane neuroses (hysteria, epilepsy, hypochondriasis, etc.)
9. Toxic insanity
10. Moral and impulsive insanity
11. Idiocy, etc.

While Morel and his colleagues were engaged on this delicate and ultimately fruitless task, several national professional organizations were pursuing similar but more modest aims. The Statistical Committee of the Royal Medico-Psychological Association produced a classification in 1882 which the Association recommended to its members for general adoption. Further revisions were produced in 1904, 1905 and 1906 before the Association finally accepted the unpalatable fact that most of its members were not prepared to restrict themselves to diagnoses listed in any official nomenclature, English or international. A similar sequence of events took place in the United States. The Association of Medical Superintendents of American Institutions for the Insane, the forerunner of the American Medico-Psychological Association and hence of the American Psychiatric Association, adopted a slightly modified version of the 1882 British classification in 1886. In 1913 what had by then become the American Medico-Psychological Association officially adopted a new nomenclature incorporating Kraepelin's concepts of manic depressive psychosis, involutional melancholia and dementia praecox. The committee responsible for producing this classification clearly understood the issues and problems involved. As they stated in their official report in 1917:

'The first essential of a uniform system of statistics in hospitals for the insane is a generally recognized nomenclature of mental diseases. The present condition with respect to the classification of mental diseases is chaotic. Some states use no well-defined classifications. In others the classifications used are similar in many respects but differ enough to prevent accurate comparisons. Some states have adopted a uniform system, while others leave the matter entirely to the individual hospitals. This condition of affairs discredits the science of psychiatry and reflects unfavourably upon our Association, which should serve as a correlating and standardizing agency for the whole country. . .' (see May, 1922).

Unfortunately the committee's clarity of vision did not suffice to ensure the achievement of its objectives. The New York State Commission in Lunacy insisted on retaining its own classification, drawn up some years before by Theodore Hoch and Adolph Meyer, and indeed continued to do so until 1968; other states and hospitals did likewise, or adopted the association's nomenclature in theory but not in practice, or declined to be bound by any nomenclature, national or local.

## The reasons for failure

To those involved in our contemporary efforts to secure agreement on the composition of an international classification, and then to persuade psychiatrists to use it rather than merely to pass resolutions adopting it, the history of these earlier failures makes sobering reading. There is a frightening familiarity to it all. The costumes and the names of the actors are different now, but as the plot unfolds it becomes clear that the characters and their roles remain much the same today as they were then. The commissions of sixty and ninety years ago saw the need for a single classification acceptable to everyone as clearly as our own expert committees, but they failed to achieve their objective for a number of cogent reasons. They found themselves forced to choose between several existing classifications, each acceptable only to its own authors; they were handicapped by ignorance of the aetiology of the conditions they were trying to classify; they were unable to agree amongst themselves whether classification should be on the basis of symptomatology, psychology, aetiology, or outcome, or a combination of all four; and they were dealing with professional colleagues who were often as disinclined to have a uniform nomenclature imposed on them as they would have been to have uniform methods of treatment imposed on them. None of these problems has melted away with the passage of time. On the other hand, with the benefit of hindsight one can see that the end of the 19th century and the early years of the 20th were a singularly unfavourable time to try to impose uniformity. In the two or three decades before Kraepelin introduced his great synthesizing concepts of dementia praecox and manic depressive psychosis all existing classifications were so obviously unsatisfactory that none could hope to command wide allegiance. And then the impact of these new concepts at the turn of the century was so great that some time needed to elapse before the disruptions they caused had subsided sufficiently for a new consensus to be capable of developing. Even in 1937, when the need for an international classification was discussed once more, this time at the Second International Congress for Mental Hygiene, it soon became apparent that there was little hope of any real consensus emerging, though the simple eight category classification proposed by the French psychiatrist Bersot was finally adopted by two countries, Portugal and Switzerland, and remained in use in both for twenty years.

Only is the last twenty five years has the situation started to improve, and it has only done so because new and more favourable influences have begun to make themselves felt. The need for an international classification is much more obvious to a generation of psychiatrists accustomed to frequent meetings with colleagues from other countries at international conferences, and who have often worked abroad themselves, than it was to their more insular predecessors whose contacts with foreign colleagues were few and far between. The necessity for international co-operation is also becoming increasingly obvious in many other spheres, political and economic as well as scientific. Increasing recognition of the importance of epidemiological data, not just for the planning of services, but also as a potential means of elucidating the aetiology of mental illness, is another important change. Until quite recently the paradigm model for research, in psychiatry as in the rest of medicine, was the detailed study of the individual. Whether attention was focused on his brain or on his mind, the strategy was essentially the same. In such an atmosphere accurate classification is desirable, but perhaps not essential. But once the need to compare one population with another is accepted, or to study the effect of environmental factors on incidence or prevalence, accurate classification becomes mandatory.

## The International List of Causes of Death

Modern attempts to produce an international classification of mental illness have developed within the context of a sustained effort by the World Health Organization to produce an internationally acceptable classification of all diseases, an attempt which has a long and distinct history of its own. Largely at the instigation of two medical statisticians, William Farr in London and Jacques Bertillon in Paris, the International Statistical Congress had, as far back as 1853, recognized the need for 'une nomenclature uniforme des causes de décès applicable à tous les pays' and had not only produced a nomenclature, but revised it at regular intervals for the next fifty years. Probably because of the obvious importance of mortality statistics to governments and public health officials, these successive editions of what came to be known as the Bertillon Classification of Causes of Death were used more and more widely, until in

1899 the International Statistical Institute urged that the task of sponsoring and revising it should be taken over by some more weighty governmental body. The French Government accordingly convened a series of international conferences in Paris in 1900, 1920, 1929 and 1938, and thereby produced four successive editions of what was now called the International List of Causes of Death.

THE 6TH EDITION OF THE INTERNATIONAL CLASSIFICATION

When the World Health Organization came into being in 1948 one of its first public actions was to produce a 6th revision of this *International List* (WHO, 1948). Renamed the *International Statistical Classification of Diseases, Injuries and Causes of Death*, this was for the first time a comprehensive nosology* covering the whole range of disease, rather than merely causes of death, and so for the first time included a classification of mental illness. In fact, Section V of this 6th revision, entitled 'Mental, Psychoneurotic and Personality Disorders', contained ten categories of psychosis, nine of psychoneurosis and seven of 'disorders of character, behaviour and intelligence', most of them subdivided further. Farr had recognized nearly a century before that 'it is evidently desirable to extend the same system of nomenclature to diseases which, though not fatal, cause disability in the population, and now figure in the tables of the diseases of armies, navies, hospitals, prisons, lunatic asylums. . . .' (Registrar General, 1856). Indeed, largely at his instigation, several of the successive nomenclatures produced by the old International Statistical Congress and the subsequent international revision conferences in Paris had included such a list, but it had never been more than a rudimentary appendage to the basic cause of death list and had never come into widespread use.

Unfortunately, although the nomenclature of ICD–6 had been unanimously adopted by the 1948 revision conference, and was duly 'recommended for use' by all the member states of the WHO, its mental disorders section failed to gain acceptance and eleven years later was found to be in official use only in Finland, New Zealand, Peru, Thailand and the United Kingdom. History was again repeating itself. Deeply concerned by this state of affairs the WHO asked an English psychiatrist, Erwin Stengel, to investigate the situation and if possible to make recommendations. His report was an impressive document and had a considerable influence on the subsequent policies of the Expert Committee on Mental Health of the WHO (Stengel, 1959).

* It may be helpful to provide some definitions here. A *nosology* is a classification of disease (from the Greek word for disease, νόσος), whereas a *taxonomy* is a classification of animals or plants. A *nomenclature* is simply an approved list of categories or titles. In order to constitute a *classification* its categories must be mutually exclusive and jointly exhaustive, and may have other formal relationships to one another as well, being arranged either in tiers (orders, genera, species, etc.) or in a hierarchy.

*Stengel's report*

The situation Stengel encountered he described as one of 'almost general dissatisfaction with the state of psychiatric classification, national and international' and the attitude of many psychiatrists towards classification, at least in its conventional forms, seemed to have become 'one of ambivalence, if not of cynicism'. Many European and North American countries had official classifications of their own, some of recent origin, others dating back to the 1930's, but none, new or old, was regarded as satisfactory by its users, or applied conscientiously and consistently by them. The United Kingdom was the only major country in which the ICD nomenclature was in official use and even here the situation was anything but satisfactory. The General Register Office published mental hospital admission rates and other morbidity data in the format of the ICD but the returns from individual hospitals from which these data were derived frequently showed a blatant disregard for the requirements of the nomenclature. The majority of depressive illnesses were listed simply as 'depression' or 'depressive illness', leaving it quite unclear whether they were to be classified as manic depressive reactions (ICD 301), involutional melancholia (ICD 302) or neurotic depressive reactions (ICD 314). The categories for psychoneuroses with somatic symptoms (ICD 315–317) were hardly used at all, and the admission rates for several other categories varied so wildly from place to place that it was inescapable that very variable meanings were being applied to the terms involved.

In the United States, Section V of the ICD was ignored completely, in spite of the fact that American psychiatrists had taken a prominent part in drafting it. Instead, a classification drawn up by the American Psychiatric Association's Committee on Nomenclature and Statistics was in widespread use, having been officially adopted by the APA and published in 1952 in a Diagnostic and Statistical Manual, known colloquially as DSM-1 (American Psychiatric Association, 1952). Although it reflected a different orientation and tradition from that of the ICD and European psychiatry, this classification was in many ways superior to its contemporaries elsewhere. It was widely available in a carefully prepared booklet, and most of its constituent categories were accompanied by working definitions or thumbnail descriptions of the syndromes concerned. Moreover, adequate publicity was given to its existence and to the need for all American psychiatrists to bring their own diagnostic predilections into line with its requirements. But in spite of this many problems remained. It was widely criticized by influential men like Karl Menninger, and widely ignored by the less influential, and the New York State Department of Mental Hygiene, now under the influential guidance of Paul Hoch, still insisted on retaining its own classification. It was also this nomenclature which Ward and his colleagues were using in the well known reliability study in which they concluded that nearly two thirds of all diagnostic disagreements between psychiatrists were due to the inadequacies of the classification, rather than to those of the interviewer or the patient (Ward, Beck, Mendelson, Mock and Erbaugh, 1962).

## The aetiological implications of diagnoses

There were, of course, good reasons why psychiatrists still found themselves unable to produce an acceptable international classification, in spite of an apparently genuine recognition of the need for one. Partly it was a matter of disenchantment with the whole subject of diagnosis and classification arising from many sources: a reaction against the sterility of earlier generations' preoccupation with nosology, growing awareness of the low reliability of routine clinical diagnoses, and a similar awareness that, no matter what categories were used, a large proportion of patients always seemed to fall between two stools, on the boundary between one syndrome and the next. But powerful feelings were involved as well. As an epidemiologist with personal experience of the situation was once driven to remark, 'at times the emotion surrounding psychiatric nomenclature. . . reaches the fanatic proportions which in earlier times surrounded debates as to how the deity should be named' (Gruenberg, 1969).

Stengel became convinced that the main reason for these strong feelings, and the resultant impasse, lay in the aetiological implications of diagnostic terms, and that it was the theoretical objections of different schools of psychiatry to each other's assumptions about aetiology which lay at the root of the problem. With some diagnoses, like psychogenic psychosis, reactive depression and conversion hysteria, these assumptions are explicit. But many other diagnoses carry with them, or are widely assumed to carry with them, implicit assumptions which may be equally potent; a diagnosis of involutional melancholia being taken to imply, for instance, that depressions of this type have a different aetiology from other depressive psychoses, and a diagnosis of schizophrenia to imply that the illness is 'endogenous' and bound to result in irreversible deterioration.

## Operational definitions

Stengel's answer to this problem, and his most important recommendation, was that all diagnoses should be explicitly shorn of their aetiological implications and regarded simply as 'operational definitions' for certain specified types of abnormal behaviour. In this he was following Carl Hempel's advice (Hempel, 1961) though for rather different reasons, Hempel having been concerned to achieve reliability and precision rather than to avoid theoretical overtones. But whatever the motive, and both are equally sound, it follows that the type of behaviour, or combination of symptoms, involved must be specified without ambiguity. If schizophrenia is to be regarded merely as an arbitrary operational label for certain rather odd ways of behaving or experiencing, without carrying any implications about their aetiology or prognosis, those ways of behaving or experiencing must be adequately described if the term schizophrenia is to have any clear meaning. Stengel does not seem to have fully appreciated this. He realized quite clearly that the sort of nomenclature he was proposing would be of little use without a companion glossary, indeed he stressed that this would need to be 'available from the beginning in as many languages as possible', but he did not seem to realize that it was not sufficient for this glossary merely to list the characteristic features of each condition. An operational definition in Hempel's sense has to specify precisely which individuals do and which do not qualify for inclusion and a thumbnail sketch of a typical patient or a list of commonly encountered symptoms does not do this. It may identify the core of the concept fairly accurately, but it fails to identify its margins. (This issue is discussed more fully in chapter 10.)

THE 8TH EDITION OF THE INTERNATIONAL CLASSIFICATION

A new edition of the *International Classification*, the 8th, was published in 1965 and came into use in 1969. [A 7th edition had appeared in 1955, but its mental disorders section was identical to that of the previous (6th) revision.] This 8th revision was a considerable improvement on its predecessor and owed much to the careful assessment Stengel and his colleagues on the WHO Expert Committee had made of the shortcomings of the 1948 nomenclature. One of the most widespread criticisms of this had been that many psychiatric illnesses could not be classified in the mental disorders section. General paralysis, for instance, was classified with other syphilitic disorders in Section I [Infective and Parasitic Diseases] and Huntington's chorea in Section VI [Diseases of the Nervous System and Sense Organs]. Section V of the new revision was made self-sufficient by creating categories within it for all psychiatric disturbances, psychotic and non-psychotic, arising on a basis of organic disease. The sections dealing with personality disorders, sexual deviations, mental retardation, alcoholism and drug addiction were all expanded and recast, and a new group of reactive psychoses was introduced to meet the wishes of Scandinavian psychiatrists. More important than these textual changes, however, was the process of international co-operation and persuasion that accompanied them. The American Psychiatric Association, in the face of considerable domestic opposition, and despite a reversion to a psychosis/neurosis terminology in place of the Meyerian 'reactions' of ICD–6, agreed to forego its independence and produce a new Diagnostic and Statistical Manual (DSM–2) based on the nomenclature of ICD–8. With the Scandinavian and German psychiatric societies also agreeing to use this new nomenclature the pendulum swung decisively. For the first time all the major contributors to the psychiatric literature, with the notable exception of France, were officially committed to using the same classification.

Unfortunately, the committee responsible for producing the nomenclature did not start work on the companion glossary that Stengel had recommended until 1967, and did not complete the task until 1972, three years after ICD–8 had come into use and seven years after its original publication. This delay greatly reduced the usefulness, and also the authority, of the new classification. On the other hand, even if it had been possible to complete the long processes of consultation and compromise involved before 1969, it may well be that opposition would have been far greater had all its implications been spelled out from the beginning. There are, after all, occasions when it is wiser to start with the thin end of the wedge. Be that as it may, two national societies, the American and the British, stepped into the breach, with the active encouragement of WHO, and produced glossaries of their own in time for the formal introduction of ICD–8 in 1969. (American Psychiatric Association, 1968; General Register Office, 1968.)

*The American and British glossaries*

Without any doubt both these glossaries have served a useful purpose and the frequency with which they are referred to in the literature is evidence that they are often used by research workers wishing to provide, or obtain, authoritative criteria for the diagnostic categories with which they are concerned. The British glossary, for example, was used by the US/UK Diagnostic Project as an arbiter of the meaning of the various diagnostic terms in the ICD–8 nomenclature, and continues to be used in the same way by the Aberdeen and Camberwell case registers. However, it is equally clear that both glossaries are unsatisfactory in many respects. Neither makes any real attempt to provide the operational definitions Hempel was advocating, or to define the global category of mental disorder with whose subdivisions they are concerned. Nor do the brief notes provided by them for each diagnostic category follow any consistent pattern. At times they list the typical clinical features of the condition, at others they merely state which other conditions are excluded. Sometimes a particular (and hypothetical) aetiology is specified, and sometimes the age and other details of affected subjects are specified, though more usually neither is mentioned. The American glossary provides more detailed guidance on the classification of organic states and the different varieties of mental retardation, and also contains a number of private subcategories not in the original international nomenclature, whereas the British glossary tends to provide fuller descriptions of typical symptom patterns in the main areas of functional illness. In some instances the two are in open disagreement. For example, in DSM–2 the category latent schizophrenia (ICD 295.5) is stated to be 'for patients having clear symptoms of schizophrenia but no history of a psychotic schizophrenic episode', whereas in the Registrar General's glossary the same category is described as being 'used to designate those abnormal states in which, in the absence of obvious schizophrenic symptoms, the suspicion is strong that the condition is . . . schizophrenia'. Another important disparity is that the British glossary defines mental retardation (ICD 310–315) in the same way as the 1959 Mental Health Act as 'a state of arrested or incomplete development of mind', thereby implying that the defect is innate and irreversible, whereas the American glossary defines it as a state of 'subnormal intellectual functioning' originating 'during the developmental period' from any of a wide variety of causes, including experiential ones, and so not necessarily irremediable (Ewalt, 1972). Both glossaries also contain more or less thinly veiled invitations to backtrack on the international agreements reached with such difficulty beforehand. In the British glossary the categories reactive depressive psychosis and reactive excitation (ICD 298.0 and 298.1) are described as being '*supposed* to be precipitated by a psychological trauma', and this revealing phrase is followed by the comment that 'psychiatrists who do not recognize this category, include this condition under 296.2'. DSM–2 is even more blatant. Both categories are placed in square brackets, implying that they are 'to be avoided in the United States or used by record librarians only'.

However, the most conspicuous failure at least of the British glossary has been its failure to make any perceptible impact on the diagnostic behaviour of ordinary clinicians. A comparison between two samples of a thousand diagnoses attributed to mental hospital inpatients in 1968 and in 1971 respectively, before and after the formal introduction of the new nomenclature and its companion glossary in January 1970, revealed almost no difference between the two (Kendell, 1973b). In 1971, over a year after the official introduction of ICD–8, only 27 per cent of diagnoses were expressed in the nomenclature of that revision, compared with 25 per cent in 1968. In both years, fully 37 per cent of all diagnoses were quite uncodable in ICD terms, either because the syndrome was not specified in sufficient detail to restrict it to a single ICD category even at the 3 digit level, or because the diagnostic term used was not recognized in the ICD nomenclature even as an inclusion term. It may well be that the inadequate publicity with which the new nomenclature and glossary were introduced is to blame for this sorry state of affairs, rather than the shortcoming of the glossary or the indifference of British psychiatrists to issues of classification, but either way it is clear that the most important task facing the Registrar General's Advisory Committee in future is the political one of persuading their colleagues to use any nomenclature at all, and to teach their students to do likewise, rather than the academic one of remedying the deficiencies of the current nomenclature. It would be interesting to know whether DSM–2 has suffered the same fate in the United States.

*The international glossary*

The final version of the WHO glossary to ICD–8 was produced as an appendix to the report of the eighth annual seminar on the standardization of psychiatric diagnosis (WHO 1973b), but it has still not been officially published and as yet few people are aware of its existence. There is no doubt that it is a significant improvement on both the American and the British national glossaries, partly because it had the benefit of users' comments on both of these, and partly because its successive drafts had been subjected to informed criticism from many different countries and even to pilot trials in some of these (e.g. Norway and the USSR). In particular, it provides more detailed guidance on the use of the organic categories (290–294) than either of the national glossaries, a less half-hearted acceptance of the reactive psychoses (298), and a breakdown of the behaviour disorders of childhood category (308) into five subcategories, including infantile autism and the hyperkinetic syndrome.

*The shortcomings of ICD–8*

It is difficult for any glossary or set of definitions to rise above the limitations of the classification to which it relates. The nomenclature of ICD–8, although undoubtedly an improvement on that of ICD–6, still has a number of serious defects. The most fundamental of these is that its constituent categories are distinguished from one another partly on the basis of symptoms and partly on the basis of aetiology. In all branches of taxonomy, theorists have almost invariably stressed the need for classification to be based on a single unitary principle though, as Stengel pointed out in 1959, where classifications of disease are concerned all those which are at all widely used in practice are based on a mixture of two or more principles, whereas those with a unitary basis have generally proved artificial and unworkable. As it happens, classifications of mental illness are generally less heterogeneous than those of other diseases because so little is known of aetiology that most conditions have to be defined in terms of their clinical features *faute de mieux*. Even so, it soon became clear that in practice the mixture of symptoms and aetiology on which ICD–8 was based was causing numerous problems. As Wing pointed out on the basis of her experience of coding the diagnoses attributed to patients on the Camberwell register (Wing, L., 1970), the fact that organic psychoses (290–294) were classified on the basis of aetiology made it impossible to distinguish between deliria, confusional states and dementias, whereas in practice clinicians were often unable to determine the aetiology of these syndromes and so only able to make such diagnoses as 'acute confusional state – cause undetermined'. Furthermore, in some cases in which aetiology was known, or at least strongly suspected, the British glossary left it unclear whether this should take precedence over symptomatology or not, whether, for instance, a schizophrenic illness precipitated by alcoholism should be classified as an alcoholic psychosis (ICD 291) or as schizophrenia (ICD 295).

*The separation of aetiology and symptomatology*

The Swedish psychiatrist Essen-Möller has long advocated a classification with separate axes for symptomatology and aetiology as the solution to this problem (Essen-Möller and Wohlfahrt, 1947; Essen-Möller, 1961, 1971 and 1973). As he repeatedly pointed out, this would make it possible to identify all cases with a given aetiology (e.g. all puerperal illnesses) regardless of their clinical symptoms, and all cases with the same syndrome (e.g. all deliria) to be similarly identified regardless of their aetiology. Such a classification would also, he considered, reduce disagreements between different schools of psychiatry by restricting disputes about aetiology to that part of the typology and, by forcing some sort of aetiological assignment to be made for every patient, lead in time to greater knowledge of aetiology. Whether or not this would really prove to be so, it is difficult to refute the logic of his main argument, or to find any other way of achieving the same end. In the last few years some encouraging signs that his advice is being heeded have begun to emerge. The report of the eighth (1972) WHO seminar on the standardization of psychiatric diagnosis contained a strong recommendation that the feasibility and acceptability of a multi-axial system of classifying psychiatric disorders should be systematically explored with a view to possibly adopting such a system in ICD–10 in the 1980's (WHO, 1973b). The draft proposals for ICD–9, due to be published in 1975, also embody an interim solution to the problems Wing described which consists in effect of having separate classifications of symptoms and aetiology for all organic states. This is to be achieved mainly by introducing two new categories for psychotic conditions secondary to organic disease, one for acute and sub acute confusional states (293), and the other for dementias and Korsakow states (294). In both cases the underlying condition, if known, would be coded separately in the appropriate section of the ICD (i.e. sections I–IV or VI–XVII), thus achieving what is tantamount to separate listing of the syndrome and its aetiology. The same would be done for childhood disorders secondary to organic disease and mental retardation.

*The psychiatric disorders of childhood*

The other serious shortcoming of ICD–8 is the inadequate provision it makes for the psychiatric disorders of childhood. Just as most classifications of mental illness in Kraepelin's day were really classifications of insanity with a few omnibus categories for non-psychotic states tacked on at the end, so most contemporary classifications are really classifications of adult illness with one or two poorly defined categories for childhood disorders added as a sort of codicil. ICD–8 is no exception to this general pattern. Apart from an elaborate classification of mental retardation, and categories for special symptoms like stammering, tics, and enuresis, only one category is provided for the behaviour disorders of childhood and even this is not subdivided.* The notes on this category (ICD 308) in the British glossary consist of one sentence, 'Only conditions which cannot be classified elsewhere should be included here', which is at least an honest recognition of its 'ragbag' function.

The WHO was not unaware of these deficiencies and the third of its annual seminars on standardization of psychiatric diagnosis was devoted to the classification of childhood disorders, and a number of child psychiatrists invited to join the parent committee for that purpose. This meeting resulted in a firm recommendation that a 'triaxial' classification with separate axes for the clinical syndrome, the child's intellectual level and 'aetiological and associated factors' be tried out and, if these trials proved successful, incorporated in the next edition of the ICD (Rutter, Lebovici, Eisenberg, Sneznevskij, Sadoun, Brooke and Lin, 1969). The fifth annual seminar subsequently made a similar recommendation for the classification of mental retardation. Rutter and his colleagues have recently reported the results of the first of these trials (Rutter, Shaffer and Shepherd, 1973). They had asked a group of twenty two British child psychiatrists to diagnose and code a series of seventeen written case histories, first using ICD–8 and then using a new triaxial system, and then to do the same thing live with ten to fifteen children newly referred to their own outpatient clinics. The results suggested that reliability was similar for both classifications, but that the triaxial one was much better at dealing with psychiatric disorders associated with mental retardation or physical illness, and at distinguishing the different clinical syndromes encountered in childhood. Perhaps of even greater significance was the fact that the participants all found the triaxial schema easy to use, even in an outpatient setting, and preferable to ICD–8. Its most obvious weakness was its handling of aetiological factors, particularly the psychosocial ones whose reliability proved to be very low. This is likely to be a persistent problem in both adult and child psychiatry as aetiology is usually unknown, and involves a complex interaction between constitutional and environmental factors, both physical and psychological, in the few instances in which it is reasonably well understood. But the difficult problems to be anticipated in this area are a reason

* The American Psychiatric Association subdivided this category on its own initiative in DSM–2, providing six subcategories (hyperkinetic reaction of childhood, unsocialized aggressive reaction of childhood etc.) each accompanied by short descriptive notes. They also added a subcategory for childhood schizophrenia and another for adjustment reactions of childhood. The WHO glossary that appeared in 1973 also provided an unofficial subdivision of ICD 308, with five slightly different subcategories including childhood autism (distinct from childhood schizophrenia), the hyperkinetic syndrome, and aggressive or destructive conduct disorders.

for, rather than against, separating aetiology from symptomatology as a separate dimension.

*Multiaxial categorization*

Once a decision has been taken to classify the syndrome and its aetiology separately the traditional 'one diagnosis' principle is breached and the way is open to create further dimensions in order to convey information about other aspects of the patient's functioning. Several people have already taken advantage of this opportunity, or succumbed to this temptation, depending on how one views it. Essen-Möller himself soon increased his two projected dimensions to three by drawing a distinction between what he called the gross syndrome (habitual state, psychosis, neurosis, or normal personality) and the specific syndrome (phobic, hallucinated, paranoid, etc.) (Essen-Möller, 1961). Rutter and his colleagues increased the three axes they started with to four by listing physical and psycho-social aetiological factors separately. Recently, Ottosson and Perris (1973) have described an even more complex classification based on four independent axes, concerned respectively with symptomatology, severity, aetiology and course. Their symptomatology axis is divided into fourteen 'symptoms in the strict sense' and twelve 'personality disturbances', and several of both are subdivided further. Severity is divided only into neurosis and psychosis, the distinction being based on 'reality evaluation', but aetiology is divided into four categories – somatogenic, psychogenic, characterogenic and cryptogenic – and course into diseases and habitual states, but with both subdivided further. From the examples Ottosson and Perris provide, it seems clear that individual patients are allowed to have several different symptoms, that each of these may have its course and aetiology charted independently of the others, and that even a single symptom may have more than one aetiology. They have, therefore, not only increased Essen-Möller's axes from two to four but also greatly increased the complexity of the system by allowing individual patients to occupy multiple positions on at least three of these axes. There is no doubt that the system is workable as it has been in regular use in both the authors' departments for several years, but it does represent a very radical departure from a single category diagnosis. In effect it is a standardized or structured formulation rather than a diagnosis and should be evaluated as such. There are, of course, considerable advantages in giving a formulation a standardized format, though there are disadvantages too, and it remains to be seen whether Menninger and the other critics of traditional diagnoses will be any more receptive to this sort of approach. However, one important characteristic of a formulation, discussed in chapter 1, is that it is needed for quite different purposes from a diagnosis and cannot be regarded as an alternative or a replacement. The implication of this is, of course, that if the sort of multi-axial schema Ottosson and Perris are advocating were to come into widespread use, and many advantages would accrue if it did, traditional diagnoses, or something like them, would still be needed as well.

Although Ottosson and Perris refer to their schema as a 'multi-dimensional classification' and other authors sometimes use the words axis and dimension interchangeably, it is important to realize that the axes discussed here are not in any way comparable to the dimensions referred to in chapter 9. Dimensions derived by principal component or factor analysis are related mathematically to one another. Although individual items often contribute significantly to several different factors, patients' scores on individual factors are independent of one another (or, if the factors are not orthogonal, the extent of their correlation is known), the distribution of scores on each factor tends towards normality, the contribution of each factor to the total variance is known, and each patient can be represented as a single locus in the multidimensional space formed by the factors. None of these properties except the last is possessed by Rutter's axes, and not even this by Ottosson's dimensions. Both these are really no more than category allocations on separate classifications representing different facets of the patient's illness. The choice and number of axes, and the number of categories allocated to each, are all determined by arbitrary decisions, and the only mathematical relationship assumed is that it is meaningful for every patient to be assigned to one or more categories on each axis. It might indeed be less confusing to refer to them as 'independent ratings' rather than dimensions. Hathaway and McKinley's MMPI and other similar scales also bear a superficial resemblance to dimensions. Indeed, the outward form of an individual's scores on Wittenborn's nine dimensions of symptomatology and on the nine psychopathology scales of the MMPI is identical. But although MMPI scale scores are all normally distributed and adjusted to the same mean and standard deviation, the original choice of nine scales rather than, say, four or twelve was arbitrary, and the choice of items contributing to each scale was determined quite independently for each by comparing criterion groups with and without the corresponding clinical diagnosis. As a result, the correlations between one scale and another are very variable and often high.

*Single v. multiple diagnoses*

For many purposes it is highly desirable for each patient to be restricted to membership of a single diagnostic category. Not only is this a fundamental principle of most classifications, and a traditional aspiration in all branches of medicine, it is also a great convenience to the statisticians responsible for the analysis of morbidity data. But clinicians frequently encounter patients whom they consider cannot be adequately described without using two or more categories. A lifelong homosexual may develop schizophrenia, a young man with a phobic neurosis may become dependent on alcohol, an elderly woman with a paranoid psychosis may develop a drug-induced acute confusional state as well, and so on. The best way of coping with this clash of interests between clinician and statistician is to allow the former to make more than one diagnosis if he wishes to, but to stipulate that one of these must be identified as the main diagnosis and the others as subsidiary, and provide clear-cut rules for deciding which should be which. In general, there are two equally arbitrary ways of doing this; to stipulate that the main diagnosis should be whichever condition is the immediate reason for referral, or requires treatment more urgently, as is done in the American glossary, DSM–2, or to provide a hierarchy of diagnoses, so that an organic psychosis automatically takes precedence over a functional psychosis, a psychosis over a neurosis, a neurosis over a personality disorder, and so forth. The latter is probably the more reliable or unambiguous of the two, and was used by the US/UK Diagnostic Project for their transatlantic comparisons.

## The hierarchy of diagnoses

In practice, clinicians only make multiple diagnoses when their patients have an organic state as well as a functional one, or an illness, neurotic or psychotic, as well as a habitual state like mental retardation or a personality disorder. They do not normally diagnose two functional psychoses simultaneously, or a neurosis and a psychosis together. The reason why this is so is that, without it ever having been formally decreed, the major psychotic and neurotic illnesses have come to be arranged in a hierarchy. First in the hierarchy come the organic psychoses. If there is evidence of organicity, perhaps a paretic Lange curve, or severe cognitive impairment, this overrides all other considerations and no symptom, psychotic or neurotic, is regarded as incompatible with that diagnosis. Next in the hierarchy comes schizophrenia. Certain symptoms are traditionally regarded as diagnostic of schizophrenia, regardless of what other symptoms may also be present, provided only that there is no question of organic cerebral disease. The 'symptoms of the first rank' which Schneider (1959) regarded as pathognomic of schizophrenia 'except in the presence of coarse brain disease' are an explicit statement of this convention, and in practice other clinicians attach a similar significance to symptoms like thought disorder and blunting of affect. The third position in the hierarchy is occupied by manic depressive illness. Even if its own characteristic features are present, organic or schizophrenic symptoms take precedence so that, for instance, patients with both schizophrenic and affective symptoms are classified as schizophrenics. On the other hand, neurotic symptoms of any kind may be present without disturbing the diagnosis, for neurotic illness comes at the bottom of the hierarchy. Among other things, this implies that neurotic depression is characterized by the absence of the characteristic features of psychotic depression, rather than by typical symptoms of its own (Foulds,

1973). In general, any given diagnosis *excludes* the presence of the symptoms of all higher members of the hierarchy and *embraces* the symptoms of all lower members. As a result, the lower down the hierarchy a diagnosis comes the more information that diagnosis conveys, though this is mainly about the symptoms the patient lacks rather than those he possesses.

It is no coincidence that the order in which diagnostic categories are arranged in the international and most other classifications is the same as their rank order in this hierarchy, for both reflect the sequence of questions psychiatrists commonly ask themselves in the course of reaching a diagnosis. Indeed the flow charts of the computer programs developed by Spitzer and Endicott (1968) and Wing, Cooper and Sartorius (1974) for converting clinical ratings into diagnoses both utilize this sequential and hierarchical arrangement, asking first whether there is evidence of organic illness, then whether schizophrenic symptoms are present, and so on.

This logical structure was first recognized and discussed in detail by Jaspers (1959) and it is still uncertain whether it is inherent in the nature of mental illness or is simply a man-made imposition. Gruenberg (1969) inclined to the latter view, regarding the 'remarkable phenomenon' he had stumbled upon essentially as a strategy adopted by psychiatrists trying to preserve the treasured single diagnosis principle in a situation in which the majority of individual symptoms were usually accompanied by a wide but variable range of other symptoms. On the other hand, Foulds (1965) has presented evidence suggesting that patients not only can, but characteristically do, exhibit the manifestations of all conditions lower down the hierarchy as well as those characteristic of their own level. In his own terminology, patients with 'non-integrated psychosis' (schizophrenia) also have integrated psychosis, personal illness and personality disorder as well, those with 'integrated psychosis' (melancholia or paranoia) also have personal illness and personality disorder, and those with 'personal illness' (neurosis) also have personality disorder. Whether or not symptoms really are distributed in the pyramidal fashion Foulds suggests, the order in which symptoms and diagnoses are arranged in the hierarchy has empirical justification. The reason why schizophrenia comes above neurotic illness in the hierarchy, for instance, is that when schizophrenic and neurotic symptoms coexist the patient's prognosis and response to treatment are determined more by the former than by the latter, so if only one diagnosis is allowable it is obviously better to regard the patient as a schizophrenic than as a neurotic.

PLANS FOR ICD–9

The current draft of the next (9th) revision of the *International Classification*, due to be published in 1975 and to come into use in 1978, embodies many minor but no really radical changes from the 8th edition (WHO, 1973b). It retains the hierarchical arrangement discussed above, but its scope is expanded in several directions, reflecting the steady increase that is taking place in psychiatry's sphere of activity. New categories have been introduced for disturbances of conduct, like group delinquency and promiscuity, which are not part of a generalized personality disorder; the section on childhood disorders has been greatly expanded; the single ICD–8 category for transient situational disturbances has been divided into a group of transient 'gross stress reactions' occurring in response to overwhelming stress and a range of less florid and longer lasting 'adjustment reactions'; and additional varieties of sexual disorder and drug abuse have been introduced, including dependence on tobacco. A detailed draft of a glossary has already been prepared and will be introduced at the same time as the new nomenclature. This is an important advance. If the various national societies can be persuaded to adopt this glossary as well as the nomenclature, instead of bringing out new editions of their own glossaries, it should in time do much to reduce existing international differences in diagnostic usage, as well as providing the bare bones of the nomenclature with some solid flesh. But despite these valuable improvements neither of the fundamental defects of ICD–8 and its glossary has been tackled. The need for separate classification of symptomatology and aetiology is only met in those limited areas in which there is an underlying or associated organic condition that can be coded in another section of the ICD, and the descriptive notes provided for each category are not much nearer to providing the clear-cut rules of application advocated by Hempel than they were in the original American and British glossaries.

It is natural for the apostles of change to feel somewhat frustrated and disappointed by this slow rate of progress. But, as Stengel pointed out is his original survey, an international classification can never be ahead of its time. It is bound to be 'conservative and theoretically unenterprising' because, like a convoy, its rate of progress is dictated by that of its slowest members. Attempts to force the pace would almost certainly lead to the breakdown of that fragile international consensus on which the whole enterprise is based and result in a return to the anarchy of the past, with every country going its own sweet way. Looking back on the progress of the last thirty years and comparing the draft of ICD–9 with ICD–6 it is evident that considerable progress has been made, both in the structure and scope of the classification and in the extent of its authority.

## The classification of depressions

Perhaps the greatest weakness of this process of evolution by committee consensus, apart from the difficulty of instituting major changes, is that it is much easier to get categories added to the nomenclature than it is to get them removed. This is so for the simple reason that national representatives are prepared to fight more strongly for the inclusion of their own favourite concepts than they are to oppose the efforts of others to do likewise. As a result there are several categories in the nomenclature which are only really used in one or two countries. The varieties of depressive illness recognized in the ICD illustrate this problem very clearly. In ICD–6 and 7 three varieties were recognized, manic depressive reactions, involutional melancholia and neurotic depressive reactions. In ICD–8 a fourth variety, reactive depressive psychosis, was added at the request of Scandinavian psychiatrists, in spite of the fact that some of those best acquainted with the problem were unconvinced of the value of any subdivision of depressive illness, and many more were unconvinced of the value of anything more than a single subdivision into psychotic and neurotic forms. In the draft proposals for ICD–9 the number of categories has risen once more, this time to five at the 3 digit level, and nine or ten at the 4 digit level. Involutional melancholia has at last dropped out, but there are still to be five subcategories of affective psychosis available for depressions, of which only three are manic depressive. Neurotic depression remains unchanged and so does reactive depressive psychosis, albeit under the title of 'other non-organic psychoses, depressive type'. However, in addition, two depressive varieties of 'adjustment reaction' have been added, one acute and the other prolonged, and an 'emotional type' of gross stress reaction as well. Finally there is a new 'depressive disorder' category, with a 3 digit code number all to itself, for 'states of depression not specified as psychotic, neurotic or reactive . . . which have no specifically manic depressive or other psychotic depressive features and which do not appear to be associated with stressful events or other features specified under neurotic depression'.

In effect, what has been done is that two or three alternative and quite incompatible ways of classifying depressions have all been included in the nomenclature simultaneously. Every country or committee member has managed to introduce, or retain, its own favoured categories and will doubtless continue to use these. As a result there will be a single international classification of depressions in name only. It is a sad commentary on the many studies of the classification of this group of illnesses that have been carried out in the last twenty years.

# 8 The Role of Multivariate Analysis in Deriving or Validating Classifications

During the last twenty years, countless attempts have been made to refine, replace or validate traditional clinical classifications of mental illness by subjecting the clinical ratings or psychometric test scores of samples of patients to various forms of multivariate analysis. By and large these attempts have not been very successful. However, because they have been and still are so numerous, because most clinicians do not possess sufficient knowledge of statistics to be able to assess them critically, and not least because those who have used these techniques have themselves often seemed unaware of their limitations, it may be worthwhile before proceeding further describing some of the statistical techniques involved. What follows is a brief non-mathematical description – written by a clinician without any formal statistical training for others in the same predicament – of the most important types of multivariate analysis, including an account of their limitations and the statistical assumptions on which they are based.

The whole domain of multivariate analysis is relatively new and developing rapidly, largely because until the advent of electronic computers the calculations involved in this branch of statistics were so tedious and time consuming that there was little stimulus to theoretical development. The rapid and enthusiastic expansion that has taken place hand in hand with developing computer technology has made a succession of complex and apparently powerful programs readily available to psychologists and psychiatrists who are unfamiliar with their theoretical basis, often before they have been adequately evaluated by statisticians themselves. This mushroom growth has multiplied the clinician's problems, preventing him ever coming to grips himself with the statistics involved, and often leaving him without a clear consensus of statistical opinion to rely on either. As a result, most clinicians, clinical psychologists as well as psychiatrists, have tended to oscillate uneasily between the two equally unsatisfactory postures of ignoring investigations based on these techniques, or accepting their confident conclusions at face value.

Although some statisticians restrict the term multivariate analysis to situations involving more than one dependent variable, in normal usage the term covers any analysis which involves multiple (i.e. more than two) interdependent variables, including those like multiple regression which only involve a single target variable. The three techniques which have been applied most frequently to problems of classification are factor analysis (including principal component analysis), cluster analysis and discriminant function analysis.

## FACTOR ANALYSIS

### PRINCIPAL COMPONENT ANALYSIS

Although the term factor analysis is often used loosely to include principal component analysis the two techniques have rather different aims in spite of their many similarities. The basic principles of both are well described by Lawley and Maxwell (1971). In a principal component analysis a set of n variates is transformed linearly into an equal number of new variates, the principal components, which are orthogonal, and hence uncorrelated. These principal components are selected in such a way that the first has maximum variance, the second maximum variance subject to remaining uncorrelated with the first, the third maximum variance subject to remaining uncorrelated with either the first or the second, and so on. They are derived (without regard for error variance in the data) from the latent roots and vectors of the correlation matrix, and the variances of the unstandardized principal components correspond to these latent roots arranged in descending order of magnitude. Although all n components are needed to reproduce accurately the original matrix of correlations, in practice the first few components usually account for a fairly large proportion of the total variance so that the later components can be ignored with little loss of information.

Essentially, therefore, principal component analysis is a means of transforming a large number of correlated variables into a smaller number of uncorrelated variables with the minimum loss of information and involves no hypotheses about the structure of the data from which the matrix was originally derived. This can best be illustrated with an example. Imagine a population of patients who have all been rated on 30 variables. The resulting matrix of correlations will contain 435 correlations (30(30—1)/2), too large a number to be handled with any ease. But after transformation by principal component analysis, the first six principal components may account for, say, 70 per cent of the original variance. If so, the total number of units of information can be reduced to 180 (6 × 30) with only a 30 per cent loss of information. The fact that the patients' scores on these principal components will tend to be normally distributed as well as being uncorrelated with one another are further advantages in many situations.

FACTOR ANALYSIS

In contrast to the method of principal components, the aim of factor analysis is to account for the covariances of the set of n variates in terms of the smallest possible number of hypothetical variates, or factors. First it has to be established that any correlation exists, that is that the correlation matrix differs from the unit matrix. If there is correlation, the next question is whether there is a single random variate f capable of accounting for the whole of that correlation. If not, then two random variates $f_1$ and $f_2$ are postulated and the partial correlation coefficients remaining after eliminating $f_1$ and $f_2$ examined, and so on, adding further variates one at a time until the remaining partial correlations between the n variates are statistically insignificant.

Although factors and principal components both take the same form, consisting, when a correlation matrix is analysed, of loadings varying from $+1.0$ to $-1.0$ on each of the original n variates, and although in practice the two types of analysis may give similar results, particularly if the original matrix is large, it can be seen that they are significantly different in intention. Principal component analysis is primarily concerned with variance and is simply a linear transformation whose main aim is one of economy. Factor analysis, on the other hand, is primarily concerned with covariance and aspires to reveal the underlying structure of the system from which the data were derived. This latter method was originally developed by the psychologists Spearman, Thurstone and Burt in the course of their attempts to elucidate the fundamental structure of human cognitive abilities. Spearman, for instance, argued from his finding that a single factor accounted for most of the covariance in a matrix of correlations between a set of intelligence tests, that performance on these was largely determined by a single attribute of general intelligence (g); while Thurstone, who obtained several different factors from a similar matrix derived from a wider range of tests, argued that these implied the existence of several different types of intelligence, his primary mental abilities. Most psychologists have continued to accept their basic premise that factors do reflect, and so reveal, the basic structure of the subject matter. Others, including many statisticians, have remained sceptical, largely because of the variety of different factor solutions that can be obtained from a single set of data and the lack of any satisfactory objective criterion for prefering one of these to the others. The number of factors obtained and their loadings are often affected considerably by relatively small changes in the size or composition of the subject sample, or in the range of tests employed. Even a single matrix can give several different solutions depending on differences in the algebra employed and whether and how the factors are rotated. As a result, although psychologists have used factor analysis extensively for nearly forty years, and in many university computer centres it now consumes a high proportion of total computing time, it still tends to be distrusted and little used outside the social sciences.

*Unjustified conclusions*

Given the aspirations of factor analysis and the enthusiasm of psychologists for the technique, it was inevitable that it would be applied to the thorny problem of the classification of mental illness. In fact it has been used for this purpose much more frequently than any other form of multivariate analysis. Many investigations have taken the following general form. The investigator obtains a set of data on a representative sample of patients, perhaps a series of clinical ratings or questionnaire responses, or a battery of psychometric test scores, and carries out a factor analysis of the matrix of correlations derived from these. Sometimes the factors are rotated to simple structure, sometimes they are allowed to become oblique (i.e. to become correlated with one another), and sometimes higher order factors are also derived. At some stage in this process the author calls a halt, usually because he is struck by the resemblance between the loadings on his factors and familiar clinical concepts, and indeed this resemblance is sometimes very striking. On this basis he then draws two conclusions: that his factors are evidence that the diagnostic concepts in question are 'genuine entities', and that the population from which his data were obtained is composed of the same number of patient types as he has factors. In fact, both these conclusions are quite unjustified as Cattell himself has recognized (Cattell, 1970). Factors and principal components are both expressions of relationships between attributes (symptoms or test scores in the context of psychiatric classification), whereas classification is concerned with relationships between individuals, and it is never justifiable to draw conclusions about the latter simply from a study of the former.

*The distribution of factor scores*

In recent years several workers have recognized this and tried to get round the problem by calculating patients' scores on their factors and looking for the bimodal or other discontinuous distributions of these that would indicate the presence of discrete subpopulations. Unfortunately, this produces many problems and is virtually doomed to failure. In the first place, although it is quite straightforward to calculate scores on principal components as these are linear functions of the original variates, factor scores cannot be calculated directly because the common factors do not fully account for the total variance of the variates and so they have to be estimated. A more serious problem, as Maxwell (1971) has pointed out, is that, as the algebra of factor analysis is based on the assumption that the original variables have a multivariate normal distribution, the factors obtained from them, being weighted sums of these, almost necessarily have a normal distribution also. Indeed, even if the variables themselves are not normally distributed, factor scores will still tend to have a normal distribution under the terms of the Central Limit Theorem ('The sum of a large number of random variables will be normally distributed if the variables are themselves normally distributed, but will also strongly approach normality almost regardless of the distributions of the variables summed'). In other words, in the unlikely event of a bimodal distribution of factor scores being obtained, the most likely explanation is not that two distinct populations of patients are present, but that the parametric assumptions on which the analysis was based have not been met. Zubin (1968) has also drawn attention to this problem and come to the same conclusion: ' . . . if we start with an assumption of homogeneity and wind up with a conclusion of heterogeneity, the only justifiable procedure is to reject factor analysis as inapplicable'. Indeed it does not require any detailed knowledge of statistics to realize that if distributions of factor scores always tend to normality, and an individual's scores on one factor are independent of his scores on other factors because they are orthogonal dimensions, there is no hope of ever constructing a typology. Most patients will obtain intermediate scores on any given factor, and even those who obtain particularly high scores on one are no more, or less, likely to score low or high on others. Indeed, even if distinct types are present, they may not be identified by factor analysis, nor will the number of factors obtained necessarily coincide with the number of types. [This issue is discussed in more detail by Torgerson (1968).]

*Q analysis*

Overall and others have attempted to circumvent this problem by using what is called inverted factor analysis or Q analysis. This is a form of factor analysis in which the original matrix is composed of correlations between pairs of individuals across all tests or ratings, instead of, as in the normal (R) analysis, correlations between ratings across all members of the population. Q correlations are in fact measures of the similarity between two individuals rather than of the degree of association between two variables. In Q analysis, the number of factors found is taken to indicate the number of types or subpopulations present, and each type is built up by assigning to it those individuals whose largest factor loadings are on the corresponding factor. The whole procedure has, however, been strongly criticized on several grounds. As Fleiss (1972) has pointed out, the correlations between the original variables (ratings or test scores) are ignored, the maximum number of identifiable types is severely restricted by the number of variables being measured, and the Q correlation, in addition to being almost uninterpretable, is a rather poor measure of similarity.

In spite of its elegance and ready availability, therefore, factor analysis is to all intents and purposes a useless tool to anyone hoping to construct a typology. It is often invaluable for delineating dimensions of symptomatology or for investigating the structure of a matrix, but under normal circumstances it is fundamentally incapable of generating anything other than dimensions.

## CLUSTER ANALYSIS

Cluster analysis is a generic term used to describe a wide variety of techniques designed to separate heterogeneous populations into relatively homogeneous subsets or clusters. Numerical taxonomy is a related term describing the use of clustering procedures in the classification of biological organisms. Although the basic idea can be traced back to the work of Zubin (1938) interest in this area has only blossomed in the last ten or fifteen years, largely because the computation involved was simply not feasible before large computers became available. The basic principles and the variety of different techniques available are well described by Everitt (1974). In principle, cluster analysis is a much more appropriate tool for tackling classification problems than factor analysis as the fundamental issue of the similarity between individuals is tackled directly. But, in spite of this, clustering techniques are beset with difficulties and pitfalls. To begin with, no formal rules can be laid down for finding clusters because a cluster is not, statistically speaking, a well defined term. The same is true of the other basic concept of the technique, that of similarity (or dissimilarity), and in practice a variety of different indices of similarity have been used – correlation coefficients, Euclidean distance, Mahalanobis' $D^2$, etc.

### Synthetic and analytic forms

In theory, the best way of deriving the most homogeneous clusters possible would be to divide the members of a heterogeneous population successively into every possible arrangement of two groups, three groups, four groups, etc., and test every such set of partitions for homogeneity. The snag is that even with quite small populations the problem is beyond the scope of the largest computers. As Lyerly (1968) has shown, even for a sample of sixteen the total number of arrangements is over ten thousand million! So resort to a variety of shortcuts, approximations, and stepwise or iterative procedures is inevitable. In practice, two basic approaches can be distinguished, the synthetic and the analytic. The synthetic approach starts by identifying the two most similar individuals in the population – similar, that is, in terms of the chosen index of similarity – and using them as the nucleus of the first cluster. Other individuals or pairs are examined subsequently to become the nuclei of further clusters, or be added to existing clusters. The sequences to be followed in this process, and criteria for inclusion, exclusion and reassignment, all have to be specified and all involve essentially arbitrary decisions. There are usually also a number of individuals left at the end who do not belong to any of the clusters and these also have to be dealt with, again in arbitrary ways. The analytic approach, on the other hand, starts by treating the whole population as one single cluster and then divides this first into two, then three, then four, and so on, seeking at each stage to make the n + 1 clusters more homogenous with respect to some chosen criterion, such as minimum 'within group' variance, than the n clusters of the previous stage. In general this second approach is preferable because it is more objective and so more easily programmed for computers, and because it ensures that every individual is assigned to one of the ultimate clusters. Clearly, if allowed to proceed indefinitely the synthetic approach would ultimately assign everyone to a single type and the analytic approach would eventually split the population into n clusters with one member each. The problem is knowing when to stop. In practice, the decision is often made on non-statistical grounds – when an arbitrary and prearranged number of clusters has been reached, or when a particular solution strikes the investigator as 'clinically meaningful'. This is because the various statistical methods that have been used in attempts to indicate the optimal number of clusters in any given set of data have proved to be rather ineffective, though Wolfe's likelihood ratio test (Wolfe, 1970) is better than most.

## The problem of establishing validity

Partly because of the large number of different techniques available, and partly because of the lack of a dependent variable, the central problem of cluster analysis is how to establish the validity of the clusters that are generated. Different programs will tend to divide any given body of data into different numbers of clusters of different composition and, as Forgy (1968) has shown, many of them will generate clusters even from data known to have a single multivariate normal distribution, i.e. not to contain clusters. It is easy enough to analyse a body of data and obtain a number of clusters whose clinical characteristics can then be described. The difficulty is to demonstrate that these groupings are superior to traditional syndromes, or to the different groups that might be produced by other clustering procedures. Strauss, Bartko and Carpenter (1973) have recently provided a salutary practical illustration of this problem. They obtained artificial sets of ratings on forty eight clinical items for twenty patients with neurotic depression, twenty with psychotic depression, twenty with simple schizophrenia, twenty with paranoid schizophrenia and twenty with mania. These data were then subjected to four different forms of cluster analysis. Each of the four gave different results and the only one to reproduce the original five clusters was a hierarchical program using correlation coefficients as its index of similarity (McKeon, 1967). Strauss and his colleagues then re-ran this program on the same data, but prepared the data beforehand in three different ways – with preliminary factoring retaining all loadings, with preliminary factoring retaining only loadings greater than +0.4, and using the raw scores themselves. Again, all three gave quite different results and only the raw scores reproduced the original five clusters.

In view of these alarming findings Strauss and his colleagues strongly advise that no cluster program should be used until it has been shown to reproduce known groups in a stable way. They also suggest a number of precautions that should be taken in any practical application, like randomly dividing the data in two to ensure that the program produces the same number and type of clusters with each, and adding or subtracting small numbers of individuals or items to or from the data and repeating the analysis to make sure that the clusters obtained are not radically altered by doing so. Some investigators have already employed checks of this kind. Lorr (1966) for instance, took the trouble to demonstrate that substantially the same psychotic clusters were obtained from several different sets of data before making any claims on their behalf and Everitt, Gourlay and Kendell (1971) demonstrated that they obtained the same four clusters from two different sets of data each subjected to two dissimilar forms of cluster analysis. But checks of this sort do no more than establish the consensual validity of the clusters concerned and in a clinical context what is really needed is evidence of their predictive validity. When an investigator produces new groupings of patients, the vital issue so far as clinicians are concerned is whether they are more homogeneous in terms of response to treatment and outcome than the traditional Kraepelinean categories. This is a much harder question to answer and so far there have only been a few preliminary attempts to do so, e.g. Paykel, 1972.

## The problem of input selection

It is likely that with developments in statistical theory and computing technology many of the shortcomings of existing clustering techniques will sooner or later be overcome. The problem of validation will remain, however, and so too will another set of fundamental problems concerning the initial choice of items. In classical Adansonian taxonomy, every feature of the organism is taken into consideration, and given equal weight with every other feature in determining the overall similarity between individuals. Sneath (1957) and others have argued that these principles should always be observed and that the temptation to select features believed to be good discriminators should be resisted – 'the history of classification abundantly shows the uncertainty of intuition in deciding what features are important'. But although this strategy may be practicable for bacteria it is not for human beings whose rateable characteristics are, literally, almost infinite. Even if it were practicable to include every feature, such a course would be likely to produce clusters based on characteristics having nothing to do with illness, like males and females, or caucasians, mongolians and negroes. Even if the field is restricted to features agreed to be associated with illness, the number of possible variables is still beyond the capacity of any cluster program, and this is so even though the number of independent variables can be reduced by transforming them into principal components beforehand.

It is clear, therefore, that some prior selection of items is inevitable and that the only point at issue is how radical this selection should be. Should, for instance, common neurotic symptoms be included in an analysis designed to identify discrete psychotic types? Most investigators have thought that they should and Lorr and his colleagues identified distinct anxious, hostile and excited types of paranoid psychosis by doing so. But, as Lehmann (1968) has pointed out, this may be no more meaningful than identifying distinct anxious, hostile and excited types of appendicitis. The dilemma confronting the investigator is that if he includes as wide a variety of items as he can, he may end up with groups which lack any practical or theoretical significance, and may also fail to detect genuinely discrete groups because the differences between these are obscured by this additional, irrelevant information. However, if he restricts his initial choice to items he expects to be relevant, he is only likely to find what he is looking for and may forfeit the chance of discovering new and unsuspected groupings. The safest course is probably to try both strategies in succession, and not to promulgate novel groups or subgroups until the new distinctions involved (as between anxious, hostile and excited types of paranoid psychosis) have been shown to be relevant to an external criterion like prognosis. Even if the elements in a new typology do have different prognoses, or are distinguished by some other external criterion, it is still advisable to compare the discriminatory power of this typology against that of a multiple linear regression using the same selection of items in order to find out whether the typology is really providing more information than the items do by themselves. The fact that the constituent groups of a new cluster analysis derived classification of depressions have different responses to, say, amitriptyline would be of only limited importance if a better prediction of response to amitriptyline could be obtained directly from patients' clinical ratings than from their cluster membership.

Finally, it must be remembered that all clustering procedures necessarily assume that every individual belongs to only one grouping. They cannot be expected to recognize patients with two separate illnesses, or to detect 'personality disorder' and 'neurotic illness' as distinct conditions if the majority of those with personality disorders exhibit the symptoms of neorotic illness also. Nor can they be expected to provide on the basis of cross-sectional data only the same groupings that longitudinal data might reveal.

## DISCRIMINANT FUNCTION ANALYSIS

Discriminant functions were introduced by Fisher (1936), elaborated by Rao (1948), and first applied to problems of psychiatric classification by Rao and Slater (1949). Essentially, their purpose is to provide optimal discrimination between two or more previously identified populations or classes, and although they were originally designed to handle continuous variables, in practice they can handle dichotomous ones almost equally well (Maxwell, 1961). The discrimination concerned may be between different diagnostic categories, or between different responses to a therapeutic agent, or in general between the members of any mutually exclusive array of nominal categories. If only a single pair of alternatives is involved, the results are identical to those of multiple regression analysis (Armitage, 1971).

Here we are concerned only with the use of discriminant functions to distinguish between different diagnostic categories. In the basic two-category situation, two populations of patients are compared, one with a clinical diagnosis of X, the other a diagnosis of Y, or non-X. Both are rated on a set of n items, each of which is believed to be relevant to the distinction between X and Y. A set of weights for these n items is then derived in such a way as to provide maximal discrimination between the two populations. This can be done in a number of ways which vary in complexity and efficiency, but a linear canonical variate which maximizes the ratio of between-group to within-group variance is the most widely used discriminant function, and with this method successive variates can be used to discriminate between more than one pair of populations. In the second stage of the analysis, a score is calculated for each patient by adding together his weighted scores on all of the n items which he exhibits. Most X patients will obtain high scores and most Y patients low scores on this function and the distance between the mean scores of the two will be maximal. If X and Y are genuinely distinct conditions their means will be well separated and the overall distribution of scores will tend towards bimodality, but if they are only variants of the same condition the majority of patients will obtain scores that are neither particularly high nor particularly low and the overall distribution will be likely to be unimodal.

If three populations (X, Y and Z) are included, the basic procedure remains unchanged, except that two canonical variates are generated instead of one; if four populations are included three canonical variates are generated; and so on, provided the number of populations does not exceed n, the number of items. In practice these additional canonical variates often contribute little to the total variance and so can be ignored. In each case, the starting point of the analysis is two or more previously identified criterion groups and it is important to appreciate that for this reason this form of multivariate analysis is only capable of testing existing classifications and not of generating new ones.

*The criterion of bimodality*

Moran (1966) and Kendell (1968a) have both suggested that a bimodal distribution of scores on a discriminant function, obtained from an unselected population and cross validated on a second population, should be the accepted criterion of validity for all diagnostic distinctions. The latter has tried, unsuccessfully as it happened, to demonstrate bimodality between psychotic and neurotic depressions, and between schizophrenic and affective psychoses (Kendell and Gourlay,

1970a and b). Fleiss (1972) has argued that this criterion is too stringent on the grounds that the joint distribution of two populations known to be distinct on other grounds may be unimodal if their means are close together. He also describes a method for estimating whether any given distribution is best accounted for by one, two, or more superimposed normal distributions. Although in the example he gives (a distribution of scores on a discriminant function between psychotic and neurotic depressions) the observed distribution was adequately accounted for by a single normal distribution, there is no doubt that his criterion is more sensitive, and therefore less demanding, than that of bimodality. Perhaps the choice between the two criteria should depend on circumstances. To the research worker intent on uncovering the basic structure of his material, Fleiss' criterion may be more attractive, though in general it will always be easier to account for an observed distribution in terms of two or more superimposed distributions than with one, simply because there are more independent variables available to juggle with. To the clinician, faced with the need to classify individuals and take action on the basis of that decision, the existence of a 'point of rarity' is likely to be an essential requirement, for the practical reasons discussed in chapter 5.

## The limitations of discriminant functions

Although they do not raise such daunting problems of validation as factor analysis and cluster analysis, discriminant procedures are not so powerful as they might appear at first sight, nor are their results always unambiguous. In the first place, although a bimodal distribution of scores on a discriminant function is strong evidence for the existence of two populations (provided the initial data were obtained from an unselected population and the bimodality holds up to cross-validation on a second set of data) failure to obtain a bimodal distribution is not evidence that two populations are not present. However many times a unimodal distribution is obtained, the possibility always remains that a different selection of items or more reliable criteria for allocating patients to the diagnostic categories concerned might have yielded a bimodal distribution. Nor do we possess a satisfactory objective criterion of bimodality. In practice it is customary to compare the observed distribution of scores with a normal distribution matched for mean and standard deviation by means of a $\chi^2$ test, and then assess bimodality visually if the observed distribution proves to be significantly non-normal. Conversely, a multimodal and significantly non-normal distribution does not necessarily indicate that two or more discrete populations are present. Experience has shown that under some circumstances this can be produced by failure to fulfil the parametric assumptions on which discriminant functions are based (Kendell and Post, 1973).

The other big problem, as with clustering procedures, is the selection of items.

These should be the best available discriminators between the diagnostic categories concerned and from a purely statistical point of view the number employed is not critical, provided it does not exceed $N-1$, where N is the number of patients in the smallest of the diagnostic groups involved. Theoretically, the addition of each extra item, up to this ceiling of $N-1$, should tend to improve discrimination and ought not to be capable of impairing it. But as Rao (1968) has pointed out, in practice, because the exact values of the parameters needed for setting up the optimum decision rule are unknown, additional items may result in a loss rather than a gain of efficiency. This creates an unwelcome element of chance, though the introduction of stepwise techniques may prove to be an effective way of dealing with the problem. These procedures usually start by selecting the single item which discriminates best on its own, add to that each of the remaining $n-1$ items in turn to find the most effective pair, then combine the remaining $n-2$ items with this pair one by one to find the best group of three, and so on, sometimes following this process of one by one addition by the reverse process of one by one subtraction. Melrose, Stroebel and Glueck (1970) were the first to use such a program on psychiatric data, though without being conspicuously successful.

It must also be appreciated that no conclusions can be drawn about the relative importance as discriminators of individual items from a comparison of their loadings on a discriminant function. The fact that item p has a loading of 0.53 whereas item q has a loading of only 0.29 does not necessarily mean that the former is a better discriminator than the latter in isolation. This is because the loadings are strongly affected by the complex correlations between all the items in the analysis and engineered simply to maximize overall 'between group' discrimination, regardless of their individual contributions, or their effects on individual patients. In practice, if a discriminant analysis is repeated after the addition or subtraction of one or two items the magnitude and rank order of the loadings of the remaining items are often altered considerably, and in ways that would have been impossible to predict from a knowledge of their individual contributions.

CONCLUSIONS

Three recurrent themes stand out in this discussion: the need to satisfy initial parametric assumptions, the lack of adequate criteria for deciding which and how many items should be used as input, and the problem of validating results. Factor analysis is based on the assumption that the material as a whole has a multivariate normal distribution and discriminant function analysis on the further assumption that the various criterion groups have equal variance/covariance matrices as well. In the case of factor analysis, the need to satisfy this requirement effectively prevents the method from being used to construct typologies or identify discrete populations. In the case of discriminant functions, failure to satisfy the requisite assumptions may result in the emergence of uninterpretable multimodal distributions as well as an overall reduction in efficiency. The second problem, that of item selection, raises a very old issue. Looking back on the various studies published in the last twenty years it is clear that many investigators, clinicians and statisticians, have had a naive, almost Baconian, attitude to the statistical techniques they were employing, putting in all the data at their disposal on the assumption that the computer would sort out the relevant from the irrelevant and expose the underlying principles and regularities, and assuming that all that was required of them was to collect the data assiduously beforehand. With hindsight it is equally clear that this approach rarely works and that, like Galileo, the investigator has to provide hypotheses as well as data. He himself has to decide intuitively which items are likely to be relevant and which are not, and whether he is looking for categories or dimensions. In short he has to have a shrewd idea of what he is looking for before he has much chance of finding it. Unfortunately when he does find what he was looking for he, and his audience, are immediately confronted with grave problems of validation. There is no easy way of validating the dimensions identified by factor analysis or the groups identified by cluster analysis and the need for a means of doing so is rendered all the more imperative by the fact that any statistician worth his salt is likely to be able, by judicious choice of patients and items, and of factoring or clustering procedures, to produce more or less what he wants to.

The purpose of these various warnings and criticisms is not to decry the usefulness to these statistical techniques, or to suggest that we were better off before they were invented. On the contrary, properly used, all three are powerful tools which are capable of making important contributions to the resolution of our classification problems. However, too many of the clinical psychologists and psychiatrists who have used them have, either by ignoring or simply by failing to understand their limitations, drawn unjustified and overenthusiastic conclusions from the results they obtained. It also has to be accepted that so far these techniques have not fulfilled the hopes that were originally placed in them, and that the few changes that have taken place in our classifications since their introduction have mostly been in response to other influences, like the advent of new therapeutic agents or the results of genetic studies. This failure, for such it must be accounted, at least by clinicians, is only partly due to the limitations of the statistical techniques themselves. All too often they have been misused, and in many cases the quality and reliability of the clinical data to which they were applied were too low for there to be any hope of worthwhile results being achieved. But even if properly used on data of adequate reliability, they are unlikely on their own to lead to the detection of new diseases, or to general agreement on the number and nature of the dimensions underlying the phenomena of mental illness.

# 9 The Choice between Catagories and Dimensions

Two alternative methods are available for expressing the relationships between different members of a heterogenous population: grouping them into a number of subpopulations, each of which is relatively homogenous in some chosen respect; or assigning them to positions on one or more axes or dimensions. Grouping into subpopulations implies the existence, or the creation, of a classification or typology consisting of a finite series of categories. Ideally these are mutually exclusive and jointly exhaustive, and the process by which individuals are allocated to the appropriate category is known as classification, or sometimes as categorization. Assignment to a position on an axis necessarily involves measurement and implies that the relationships between different members of the population, defined by their relative positions on the axis or axes, are quantitative and linear.

Classifications are much more widely used than dimensional systems. Indeed the structure of our language, and of all verbal thinking, is based on classification. The words we use to describe objects, animate and inanimate – cow, star, apple, proton or fairy – all denote categories and the descriptive use of any of these nouns implies that the object we are referring to belongs to this category rather than to any of the other categories in the same array; it is not a horse, a planet, a pear, a neutron or an elf. There are, however, a few situations in everyday life where categorization has been replaced by the recognition of a dimension, but this has only occurred in situations where an appropriate measuring instrument is available, and where it is recognized that the distribution of individuals along the relevant scale is continuous rather than discontinuous. Height and intelligence are obvious examples. As soon as suitable instruments for measuring height became available we stopped describing people simply as tall or short and began to say how tall they were, three and a half cubits, or 174 centimetres. Similarly with intelligence. After the invention of the intelligence quotient by Binet we stopped describing people simply as clever or stupid and began defining how intelligent they were by means of this IQ. It is worth noting, though, that in everyday life there are no dimensional systems involving more than one dimension. This is probably because, while unidimensional relationships can still be adequately portrayed by words, multidimensional ones can only be described effectively in algebraic or geometric terms.

In principle, then, two alternative methods are available for describing the relationships between one patient and another, and between patients and non-patients. Either they can be classified into different types of 'disease', or they can be allocated to loci on one or more dimensions. The traditional method is that of classification into diseases, partly because this is the way in which Man has always arranged his subject matter in any area of enquiry, and partly because of the close historical relationship between medicine and the biological sciences, and the obvious advantages botany and zoology derived from the development of detailed tiered classifications of animals and plants into species, genera and orders in the 18th and 19th centuries.

## Wittenborn's dimensions of psychosis

However much they might disagree about the number and content of individual categories, most physicians have continued to assume without question that some sort of classification was as appropriate to the domain of mental illness as it was to physical illness or zoology. A few psychiatrists have questioned this assumption from time to time, but the suggestion that a dimensional representation would be more appropriate has come mainly from psychologists. Wittenborn and his colleagues in Connecticut developed an elaborate dimensional system for psychotic illness over twenty years ago with the explicit intention of 'supplanting the usual descriptive diagnosis. . . not only for research purposes, but for practical purposes of clinical description' (Wittenborn, Holzberg and Simon, 1953). Their nine dimensions of symptomatology were derived by factor analysis from clinical ratings on fifty-five 4 point scales from over 800 patients. They carried out duplicate analyses with data from separate series of acute and chronic psychotics and provided tables for converting patients' scores on their fifty-five scales into positions on the nine dimensions. It was an impressive study, particularly as their factor analyses were done by hand before computers were available, and although their dimensional system was never widely used it had a considerable influence on later workers like Lorr and Overall. [It is, of course, somewhat illogical to assume that differences within the realm of psychotic illness are best represented by a dimensional system, while at the same time, by the act of studying psychotic illness in isolation from other forms of mental illness, assuming that psychosis itself is a valid category.]

EYSENCK'S ARGUMENT IN FAVOUR OF DIMENSIONS

Although little of his own work has been concerned with patient populations, Eysenck is probably the foremost advocate of a dimensional representation of mental disorders. His views are well known and influential, particularly with other psychologists, and also alien in many ways to medical tradition. For all these reasons they deserve to be described and examined in detail. The description which follows, and the quotations it contains, are taken mainly from the opening chapter of the first (1960) edition of his *Handbook of Abnormal Psychology*, though he has expressed similar views in other places, before and since.

Like many other people, Eysenck is dismayed by the low reliability of psychiatric diagnoses, but unlike the majority of the psychiatrists who have concerned themselves with the problem, who have directed their efforts toward improving reliability, he became convinced at an early stage that an entirely new system of representation was necessary. 'No improvement is likely to occur until the basis of the present method is changed and more modern methods substituted. . .' This conviction seems to owe as much to his belief that the medical concept of disease assumes that every diagnostic category is a discrete entity with its own distinct cause, and to the inappropriateness of such assumptions to the field of mental disorder, as to pessimism about the possibility of improving diagnostic reliability, and the way in which he seeks to achieve his objective is simple and straightforward. After observing that 'the term psychiatry does not denote any meaningful grouping of problems or subjects of study' he goes on to suggest that the territory in question should be divided into a small part 'dealing with the effects of tumours, lesions, infections and other physical conditions' and a larger behavioural part 'dealing with disorders of behaviour acquired through the ordinary processes of learning'. The former would remain the territory of physicians, but the latter would be transferred to psychologists who would discard all notions of categories of disease so as to 'clear the field and disabuse the minds of research workers of outmoded and erroneous notions'. Instead would be substituted a dimensional representation based on the three dimensions identified by him as neuroticism, psychoticism and introversion/extroversion.

## The complication of professional rivalry

It will be apparent to the reader that this proposal involves the elimination of psychiatrists as well as of medical concepts of disease from the field of mental disorder, and that the views of psychiatrists and psychologists on the relative merits of categorical and dimensional schemata are likely to be coloured by their recognition of this implication. This confusion of what was already a difficult issue by professional rivalry between psychiatrists and psychologists makes it difficult for all concerned to consider the issue dispassionately, but it is probably better to face this aspect of the problem at the outset than to try to ignore it. It would, however, be misleading to see the controversy between the advocates of categories and dimensions as a clear-cut difference of opinion between psychiatrists and psychologists. Jung and Kretschemer both espoused an explicitly dimensional view of mental illness. In more limited ways the author has done so too, and so has Strauss (1973), while Lorr, who has devoted as much time and thought to classification as any psychologist, has consistently preferred a typology to any dimensional system.

At the risk of oversimplification, Eysenck's argument can be broken down into a series of six propositions:

1. Psychiatric diagnoses are unreliable and part of the reason for this is that boundaries are being imposed where none exists *in re naturae*.

2. Numerous factor analytic studies have failed to reveal any evidence of the clustering assumed by the disease model. Distributions of factor scores are almost invariably continuous and individuals tend to have scores on all factors, not just on one.

3. The medical concept of disease assumes that diseases are qualitatively distinct conditions, each with its own unique cause. These assumptions are both inappropriate and harmful where mental disorders are concerned and can probably only be avoided by explicitly abandoning the whole idea of disease.

4. By means of a statistical technique known as criterion analysis it is possible to decide whether mental illness as a whole, or psychosis and neurosis separately, are qualitatively distinct from normality, or whether they are graded traits present to varying extents throughout the normal population.

5. The results of criterion analysis, and other experimental studies, strongly suggest that psychosis and neurosis are both graded traits present to greater or lesser extent in the whole population, but distinct from one another.

6. A dimensional system of representation (based on the three dimensions of psychoticism, neuroticism and introversion/extroversion) is therefore necessary, for both theoretical and practical purposes.

Let us examine these six propositions one by one. It is certainly true that psychiatric diagnoses are often unreliable, sometimes alarmingly so, though it has also been demonstrated that with adequate training this is not inevitable. The possibility that an absence of genuine boundaries or points of rarity between one syndrome and another is an important cause of unreliability is also entirely plausible. The matter will not be debated further here as it has already been discussed in detail in chapter 3.

The other five propositions are all rather more questionable. The statement that factor analytic studies have consistently failed to reveal any evidence of clustering is perfectly true, but this is an inevitable result of the assumptions on which factor analysis is based and cannot be regarded as evidence that clusters do not exist. Factor scores always either have, or tend to have, normal distributions, for two very good reasons. The algebra of factor analysis is based on an assumption that the original variables have a multivariate normal distribution and the factors obtained from these, being weighted sums of them, must be expected to have a normal distribution also. Even if the variables themselves are not normally distributed factor scores will still tend to be so under the terms of the Central Limit Theorem. Similarly, the fact that individual patients often obtain high scores on several different factors, while others score highly on none, is an inevitable result of the fact that successive factors are orthogonal and the scores on each normally distributed. This issue is discussed in more detail by Maxwell (1971) and in chapter 8 but in essence factor analysis is only capable of producing dimensions and no significance can be attached to its failure to do otherwise.

### '*Medical models*' old and new

Eysenck's criticisms of the medical concept of disease had some justification when they were first made in the 1950's, though even then significant changes were taking place, and now, twenty years later it has changed out of all recognition. There can be very few contemporary physicians who still regard diseases as distinct entities each with its own cause. This was, of course, the dominant concept of disease in the 19th century and for some time thereafter. It owed its long ascendancy to the discovery of causal organisms for infections like syphilis and tuberculosis and of a specific cellular pathology for others like Bright's disease, amyloidosis and the neoplasms and, like other fruitful concepts in other branches of science, it eventually outlived its usefulness and was only reluctantly abandoned. It first came under criticism in the 1930's from psychiatrists like Adolph Meyer who were distressed by its mechanistic implications and then, more significantly, from Cohen (1943) who argued cogently that disease was no more than 'deviation from the normal. . . by way of excess or defect' and so prepared the way for the explicitly statistical concept which was to follow. The crucial development, and the death knell of the 'disease entity' concept, was the demonstration by Pickering and his colleagues in the 1950's that essential hypertension was a graded characteristic dependent on polygenic inheritance and shading insensibly into normality (Oldham, Pickering, Fraser Roberts and Sowry, 1960). This unequivocal demonstration that a major illness, familiar to every practising physician, was simply the end of a continuous biological distribution like height or intelligence quickly led to a radical change in physicians' ideas about the relationship between health and illness, and also about the cause of illness. It is now almost a generation since any research worker has regarded himself as engaged on a search for the cause of cancer or coronary artery disease. He is all too well aware that the final clinical picture of any disease is the result of a complex interaction between probabilistic events occurring on several different levels – occupational, dietary, genetic, social and psychological – and therefore restricts himself to a study of 'at risk factors' and their interaction with one another rather than searching for causes. Indeed the word cause is not even mentioned by Scadding in his now classical papers on the nature of diagnosis (Scadding, 1963 and 1967). In short, the assumptions inherent in the medical concept of disease are no longer so pernicious as they were twenty or thirty years ago, or as many psychologists and social scientists still believe them to be. The only assumptions involved in Scadding's definition are that the individual's behaviour is statistically abnormal, and that he is at a 'biological disadvantage' as a result, and both of these are manifestly true at least where the functional psychoses are concerned. To the contemporary medical research worker, if not to every practising clinician, diseases are little more than convenient working concepts based on a variety of different defining criteria, anatomical, physiological or behavioural, and liable to change their defining characteristics, or even to be abandoned altogether, with advances in knowledge.

*Criterion analysis*

The next two stages in Eysenck's argument both concern his technique of criterion analysis and are the crucial ones in the sense that, if they could be shown to be true, his final conclusion in favour of a dimensional representation would be established whether the three previous propositions were true or not. Criterion analysis is an attempt to provide factor analysis with an objective means of testing the validity of the factors it generates; of testing that is, whether they are genuine dimensions present as graded traits in every member of the population, or whether the relationships they express are only exhibited by a small and finite subpopulation. Its rationale is described in detail by Eysenck (1950) and its algebra by Lubin (1950). The easiest way of describing it is probably to describe an example of its application, and the obvious example to use is the one with which we are concerned at this moment, the question of whether psychoticism is a graded trait present to greater or lesser extent in all mankind, or whether it is something peculiar to psychotics.

A number of tests of the trait in question (psychoticism, in this instance) are administered to two populations, one possessing the trait and the other lacking it, e.g. psychotics and non-psychotics. The correlations between the test scores of the population *lacking* the trait (i.e. the non-psychotics by themselves) are then subjected to factor analysis and the resulting factors rotated into maximum correlation with a 'criterion column' consisting of the biserial correlations of the same tests with a diagnosis of psychosis when administerd to both populations, psychotics and non-psychotics, together. If the correlation between the criterion column and the first factor is high, then the trait in question must be present to some extent in the population supposedly lacking it, e.g. psychoticism must be present in non-psychotics. The trait must therefore be a graded one and the difference between the two populations quantitative rather than qualitative.

In practice Eysenck did this by administering a battery of fifteen psychological tests, yielding between them some sixty five different scores, to fifty psychotic depressives, fifty schizophrenics and 100 Army conscripts serving as normal controls (Eysenck, 1951). From the sixty five test scores available twenty were selected for the criterion analysis, mainly on the basis of discriminating significantly between the psychotic and control populations. The criterion column was constructed from the biserial (tetrachoric) correlations of these twenty tests with psychosis, and factor analyses were carried out separately on the intercorrelations of the test scores of the normal and psychotic groups. Each yielded two significant factors and the correlations between the first and second factors of each were high ($+0.87$ and $+0.77$ respectively), demonstrating that the pattern of intercorrelations in the control population was very similar to that in the psychotic population. The correlations between the criterion column ($C_{n,p}$) and the rotated first factor from the normal population ($F_n$), and the corresponding rotated first factor from the psychotic population ($F_p$), were also high ($+0.90$ and 0.95 respectively).

*Psychoticism as a graded trait*

Eysenck has always regarded this as strong evidence that psychotics form a continuum with normal mental states, but before accepting this conclusion at face value it behoves us to consider the limitations of criterion analysis, and other possible explanations of his findings. A crucial assumption made in criterion analysis is that the initial identification of subpopulations exhibiting and lacking the trait in question is accurate, because it is clear that if, to return to the present example, the 'normal' population contains a significant number of psychotics, this will tend to produce a similar pattern of intercorrelations between test scores in both populations. Another important shortcoming, pointed out by Eysenck, is that there is no statistical means of deciding whether the correlation between the criterion column and the rotated factor is high enough to be significant. However, neither of these limitations seems important in this instance. From the way in which the psychotic and normal control groups were obtained it is unlikely that there was any appreciable misclassification between the two, and the correlation of $+0.90$ between the criterion column and the rotated factor ($F_n$) is surely high enough to put it beyond the need of formal significance testing. We must conclude, therefore, that Eysenck is justified in claiming to have established that continuity exists between his psychotic and normal populations, *but only in those respects with which the original test battery was concerned.* It does not follow that a similar continuity would necessarily be found with a different selection of tests.

The battery of tests from which the final selection was made included a variety of different tests of comprehension, memory, perseverance, motor speed and verbal fluency, many of them extremely simple and probably chosen mainly for their brevity and ease of measurement. The twenty tests selected included, for instance, a test of how long the subject when seated could, or would, hold his leg in the air without allowing it to touch another chair; a test of how well he could draw from memory a circle with the same diameter as a half crown; and a test of how *long* he could take to write the word YEAR. None of them bore any close resemblance to the means used by clinicians to distinguish between psychosis and normality, or had been shown to be a more effective discriminator than these traditional methods. They had, to be sure, been chosen because statistically significant differences had been obtained on them between the normal and psychotic criterion groups, but it is easy to over-rate the importance of this. As Meehl (1967) has pointed out, with large enough samples everything eventually tends to correlate significantly with everything else and the only point at issue is whether these correlations are positive or negative. With sample sizes of a hundred, most tests of any kind would be likely to show significant differences between psychotic and normal populations, particularly if, as here, no attempt was made to match them on other variables like age, sex, education and intelligence.

Eysenck himself was aware of this problem, and originally said that his conclusions 'should not be taken as in any way definitive' as different results might be obtained with a different selection of tests. Unfortunately, the issue has not been clarified any further in the twenty years that have since elapsed. With very few exceptions, other authors have neither used nor even commented upon Eysenck's method of criterion analysis and in a recent review (Eysenck, 1970) the only other evidence he was able to offer in support of his view that psychoticism and neuroticism are graded traits susceptible only to dimensional representation were a series of canonical variate analyses comparing the test scores of populations of neurotics, psychotics and normals (Lubin, 1951; S. B. G. Eysenck (1956) and H. J. Eysenck (1955) and a genetic study by Cowie (1961). The three canonical variate studies all produced two significant latent roots, which in general terms is good evidence that more than two populations are present, and Cowie's study demonstrated that the children of psychotic parents are no more neurotic than those of normal parents. In each case this is evidence that the difference between neurosis and psychosis is not simply a matter of severity, but is irrelevant to the primary issue of whether either is a graded trait susceptible only to dimensional representation or whether, on the other hand, it is qualitatively different from normality, and therefore best represented by a typology.

*The relationship between 'psychoticism' and psychosis*

The fact that psychotic patients resemble other people in many important respects, and that their performance on a wide range of psychological tests overlaps with that of normal populations, is beyond dispute. What is disputed by clinicians is that this is the end of the matter and that a typology is for this reason inappropriate. If the test battery Eysenck used for his criterion analysis studies, or the items contributing to his psychoticism dimension, had contained the accepted discriminators between psychosis and normality, or had been shown to be superior to these, he would be on much stronger ground in advocating a dimensional system. But in neither case was this so.

It is true that Eysenck's 'psychoticism' is a graded trait on which several populations of psychotics have been shown to obtain significantly higher scores than normals. But this does not prove that madness is a graded trait, or indeed that 'psychoticism' has anything much in common with the clinical concept of psychosis. A naive observer examining the loadings of the psychoticism factor on the items of the PEN questionnaire would be more likely to assume that it represented a personality trait of callousness than to suspect that it measured the essence of madness. Nor would he be surprised to find, as the Eysencks have found themselves, that criminal populations, both male and female, score just as highly on P as people with acute psychoses (Eysenck and Eysenck, 1970). Although the relationship between crime and psychiatric abnormality is complex and much debated, there is no doubt that the great majority of criminals are not psychotic and never become so. Moreover, it has recently been shown that neurotics and normals may also obtain P scores as high as those of psychotics, emphasizing further that 'psychoticism' is a misleading title (Davis, 1974; McPherson, Presly, Armstrong and Curtis, 1974). Whether or not it is justifiable to regard it as an independent dimension of personality, the available evidence does not warrant its identification as a measure of psychosis, actual or potential.

THE ARGUMENT IN FAVOUR OF CATEGORIES

If one weighs up the evidence in favour of a dimensional representation of mental illness one is forced to conclude that Eysenck and his allies have not yet proved their case. On the other hand, their evidence is sufficiently persuasive to require that their arguments be taken seriously, particularly as the evidence in favour of a categorical classification is equally unsatisfactory.

*The search for discontinuities*

At present, there is little convincing evidence that the boundaries we have drawn between one syndrome and another lie at genuine 'points of rarity', i.e. that inter-forms between adjacent syndromes are less common than patients exhibiting the uncontaminated symptoms of one or other syndrome. The frequency with which clinicians are driven to employing such labels as schizoaffective psychosis, borderline psychosis, anxiety depression, and pseudoneurotic schizophrenia, the widespread evidence that different schools of psychiatry draw the boundaries between one syndrome and another in different places, and the generally low reliability of psychiatric diagnoses all suggest that syndromes merge into one another without natural boundaries in between. Roth and his colleagues in Newcastle have searched persistently for evidence of discontinuities in the distribution of symptom patterns and claim that by applying discriminant functions to clinical ratings it is possible to demonstrate the existence of genuine boundaries between psychotic and neurotic depressions (Carney, Roth and Garside, 1965) and also between depressive illnesses and anxiety states (Gurney, Roth, Garside, Kerr and Schapira, 1972). Other authors, however, have failed to confirm the first of these claims (Kendell and Gourlay, 1970a; Post, 1972) and the latter has yet to be either confirmed or refuted. Prusoff and Klerman (1974) have demonstrated that anxiety states and depressive neuroses are sufficiently different for the attempt to distinguish them to be worthwhile on empirical clinical grounds, but not that there is any point of rarity between them. Similarly, the many attempts to demonstrate a boundary between schizophrenia and schizophreniform psychoses seem to have ended in failure (Garmezy, 1968). It is not even clear that there is any natural discontinuity between schizophrenia and the affective psychoses, though this is probably the area in which the chances of demonstrating discontinuity are highest (Kendell and Gourlay, 1970b).

*Cluster analysis*

Studies based on cluster analysis of clinical ratings have been somewhat more successful, though they have to be interpreted cautiously in the light of the limitations of these techniques discussed in the previous chapter. On the basis of extensive analyses of current mental state (IMPS) ratings of large populations of psychotic patients, Lorr and his colleagues have identified nine 'psychotic types' which do seem to be stable from one patient population to another (Lorr, 1970). However, only about 60 per cent of any given sample of patients can be allocated with confidence to one of the nine, and only seven of them are present in both male and female populations. Similar evidence for the existence of genuine clustering is provided by Everitt, Gourlay and Kendell (1971). These authors subjected clinical ratings from two different series of patients, one English and one American, to two different forms of cluster analysis. Both patient populations consisted of 250 consecutive admissions to a psychiatric hospital and the ratings were derived partly from a structured mental state examination and partly from a semi-structured history. All four analyses produced separate clusters identifiable with the manic and depressive phases of manic-depressive illness, with acute paranoid schizophrenia and, somewhat less convincingly, with chronic or residual schizophrenia. But is spite of the presence of a substantial number of patients in both series with non-psychotic diagnoses none of the four analyses yielded a cluster identifiable with depressive or other neuroses, with personality disorder or with alcoholism. Two other cluster analysis studies of depressive illnesses alone, by Pilowsky, Levine and Bolton (1969) and Paykel (1971), also yielded clusters identifiable with endogenous or manic depressive depression, though in Pilowsky's study the correspondence between clinical diagnosis and cluster membership was hardly very impressive.

It appears, therefore, that the advocates of both dimensional and categorical systems are both able to point to some fairly cogent evidence in support of their respective positions, but neither has a strong enough case to put the matter beyond dispute or to dispose of the other. This suggests that it might be appropriate to consider the different strengths and weaknesses of the two before trying to choose between them.

PROS AND CONS OF DIMENSIONS

The main advantages of dimensional representation are that there is no loss of information, and maximal flexibility is preserved. Consider, for example, the advantages of an intelligence quotient over a 'cleverness classification' with two categories clever and stupid, or three categories clever, normal and stupid. Two individuals with IQ's of 160 and 120 would both, presumably, be allocated to the clever category, but this would involve losing sight of what in many situations would be an important difference between them. Similar considerations apply at the other end of the scale, and indeed at any point along it. Secondly, a distribution of IQ's can always be converted to any number of categories as occasion demands and the boundaries of these moved up or down the scale at will. But if the members of a population are all assigned to one of the three categories clever, normal and stupid to begin with, this cannot subsequently be changed to four categories or reduced to two, except by lumping together two of the existing groups, nor is there any possibility of converting them to a dimension.

A further important advantage of dimensions is that they do not distract attention from the atypical in favour of the typical, or distort people's perception of individuals lying near the boundary between two adjacent categories. As Engle (1963) has pointed out, one of the most serious drawbacks of categorical classifications is the way in which they cause individuals who seem to lie halfway between two diseases, or between a disease and a healthy state, to be overlooked or not reported. Patients exhibiting a combination of schizophrenic and manic depressive symptoms illustrate this problem very clearly. Time and again they are either put on one side and studies confined to typical schizophrenics or manic depressives or, if they are included, one or other component of their symptomatology is ignored or minimized. The exployment of a typology, in other words, leads us to expect, and so to perceive, our patients as fitting neatly into one or other of its categories whether or not they do so in reality.

There are, however, a number of disadvantages to dimensional systems. As said before, any system involving more than a single dimension can only be handled geometrically or algebraically and if there are more than three only the latter is possible. [Scores on multiple dimensions can, of course, be represented quite easily as a list of scores all adjusted to the same mean and standard deviation, or portrayed visually as a histogram. This is commonly done with MMPI scores and with the dimensional system developed by Wittenborn, Holzberg and Simon (1953).] This is not necessarily a defect, but it does mean that those using the system must have a greater familiarity with mathematics than is possessed by most contemporary physicians, and particularly by psychiatrists. A more fundamental problem is that ultimately dimensional systems usually have to be reduced to categories before the information they contain can be utilized. It may be of considerable theoretical interest to know that the correlation between response to ECT and a particular dimension of depressive symptomatology is $+0.71$, but the practical question one is interested in is how likely are patients lying between points x and y on this dimension to respond to ECT. In fact, most scientific statements are concerned with populations rather than with linear distributions or individuals and once a population has been defined, even if this is done in terms of scores on one or more dimensions, a category has been created. It may also be significant that most of the advocates of a dimensional representation of disease are essentially theoreticians. Those responsible for day to day decisions about the management of individual patients have usually found themselves forced to use some sort of typology, whether or not they have acknowledged doing so.

PROS AND CONS OF TYPOLOGIES

Perhaps the biggest advantage of categorical systems is the ease of description and conceptualization they provide. A description of a typical member of a category provides a simple and easily remembered means of defining, and subsequently of recognizing, the essence of that clinical concept, and of the essential differences between it and other categories, even if it does not make it clear precisely how typical other patients have to be to qualify for membership. It is also difficult to ignore the fact that classification is the norm in the great majority of the areas of study Man has defined for himself and is inherent in the structure of all his languages. Moreover, the history of the biological sciences in general, and of medicine in particular, provides innumerable examples of the importance of classification, or perhaps one should say of accurate classification, as a precondition for advances in understanding. The discovery of a specific pathology for general paralysis by Noguchi, and a specific treatment by von Jauregg, would hardly have been possible if the syndrome of general paralysis had not first been distinguished from other forms of insanity by Esquirol. Nor is it easy to visualize how the mechanism of oedema formation in heart failure could have been elucidated without a prior classification of dropsy into renal and cardiac forms. It is not true, either, as some critics have suggested, that classification is dangerous because it imposes a premature rigidity on the subject matter. Inappropriate or rigid classifications owe these characteristics to the theoretical considerations inspiring them rather than to the act of classification per se. Indeed many classifications are in a state of more or less continuous flux with new categories constantly being introduced and old ones discarded in response to new ideas and observations.

Most of the disadvantages of categorical systems have already been alluded to and depend to a large extent on whether or not the boundaries between adjacent categories are drawn at genuine points of rarity. If they are problems are few, but if they are not and a high proportion of patients lie close to the boundaries between adjacent categories, numerous difficulties arise. The reliability of the system is low because different observers cannot agree which category such borderline patients should be allocated to, and because they are an embarrassment they are often ignored, or their characteristics distorted by halo effects. There is also an innate tendency to reification. Because the category and those attributed to it has a name, it acquires a shadowy 'existence' of its own, and it eventually comes to be assumed that its members must differ in some fundamental way from members of the other categories in the typology, and also that there is a fundamental difference between the mentally ill as a whole and normal people.

Another problem involved in using a typology in a situation in which no discontinuities or 'points of rarity' have been demonstrated is that it is not immediately clear where, or on what principles, the boundaries should be drawn between adjacent categories, or indeed how many categories should be established. A point of rarity has a double significance. It demonstrates the presence of an entity, and also identifies where its boundary lies and the aphorism about the art of classification consisting in learning to carve nature at the joints illustrates the dilemma that arises if no joints are to be found.

### Outcome as a diagnostic criterion

We have already agreed (see chapter 3) that the usefulness and validity of a classification are largely dependent on the strength of its prognostic and therapeutic implications. This suggests that boundaries should be placed in such a way that categories are as homogeneous as possible with respect to prognosis, or as a statistician would put it, so that the ratio of 'between group' to 'within group' variance is maximal in this respect. However, prognosis and treatment response* must not be allowed to become part of the defining criteria of a diagnostic category themselves. There is a crucial difference between defining an illness in terms of symptoms A, B and C, each of which has been shown to be associated with good prognosis, and making good prognosis itself part of the defining characteristic of the illness. The latter is unacceptable for two very good reasons. If diagnosis is to be of any use in determining treatment, it must be based on information available prior to the institution of treatment, rather than on data which can only become available subsequently. And it is in any case illegitimate to use as a defining characteristic something which is also being used as a criterion of validity.

The history of psychiatry contains many examples of failure to appreciate this distinction. Kraepelin used lifetime prognosis as his main criterion for distinguishing between dementia praecox and manic depressive psychosis. Because of this many people, including himself initially, were dismayed when some patients diagnosed as having dementia praecox recovered completely, while others regarded as having manic depressive psychoses failed to do so, and reacted by assuming that the initial diagnoses must have been wrong. Perhaps in some cases it was, but only if the patients' original symptoms had been misjudged, not simply because their illnesses took an unexpected course. When patients with the symptoms of dementia praecox recovered the conclusion that should have been drawn was that the prognosis of that condition was less homogeneous than had originally been hoped, not that the diagnosis in those patients was wrong. A diagnosis can legitimately be changed if the patient's symptoms change, and the defining symptoms of a diagnostic category can be altered in an attempt to reduce the proportion of patients with atypical prognoses. However, the diagnosis in an individual must never be changed because the course or response to treatment of his illness is atypical or unexpected. If a patient given a diagnosis of schizophrenia recovers completely that may be a reason for taking a close look at his original symptoms, or even for suggesting stricter criteria for a diagnosis of schizophrenia, but it is not in itself a justification for questioning or changing the diagnosis in that patient. The same applies to patients with involutional melancholia whose illnesses recur in the senium, or alcoholics who revert to social drinking.

THE CHOICE BETWEEN CATEGORIES AND DIMENSIONS

In attempting to choose between categorical and dimensional schemata in any given situation, it is important to realize that in principle both are available. As Cattell (1970) has said, 'the description by attributes and the description by types must. . . be considered face and obverse of the same descriptive system. Any object whatever can be defined either by listing measurements for it on a set of

* Treatment response, of course, is simply prognosis under certain specified conditions.

attributes or by sequestering it to a particular named category.' It is therefore almost meaningless to ask which is right. The appropriate question is always which is more useful or more appropriate, and the answer may well vary with the purpose in mind. It may also depend on the stage of development the subject has reached. As Hempel (1961) has pointed out, most sciences start with a typology and dichotomous present/absent distinctions, but often replace these later on with dimensions as more accurate measurement becomes possible.

*Psychotic illness*

At the present time the advantages of, and arguments for, a typology are stronger in the realm of psychotic illness than they are for neurotic illness and personality disorder. In these areas the arguments for a dimensional system are considerably more convincing, and it may well be, as Torgerson (1968) has suggested, that we may eventually be driven to use a combination of the two. Briefly, the argument for retaining a typology for psychotic illnesses is this. Kraepelin's original division of the functional psychoses into distinct affective and schizophrenic groups is almost the only aspect of our existing classification that has never been seriously challenged. There is evidence from cluster analysis studies of stable clusters of patients identifiable with these traditional syndromes, and evidence from cross-cultural studies that these syndromes occur in such a wide range of different cultures that they are probably universal (WHO, 1973a). There is incontrovertible evidence that genetic factors are involved in the transmission of both schizophrenic and manic depressive illness, and suggestive evidence that, at least in some families, manic depressive illness is transmitted by a sex-linked gene (Reich, Clayton and Winokur, 1969; Mendlewicz, Fleiss and Fieve, 1972). This last consideration is particularly important because, if confirmed, it is evidence of a qualitative or present/absent difference between the disease genotype and normal people, and this would be an almost irresistible argument for categorical representation. In addition, the reliability of our present classification is much higher for psychotic diagnoses than for neuroses and personality disorders, and its low reliability overall is largely the result of the problems caused by the latter. There are also stable differences in long term prognosis and response to therapeutic agents like ECT, tricyclic antidepressants, phenothiazines and lithium salts between manic, depressive and schizophrenic populations, and facts such as these, though not evidence that mania, depression and schizophrenia are distinct entities, are good evidence of their utility as clinical concepts.

The weaknesses in Eysenck's argument that psychoticism is a graded trait have already been discussed. It is also worth noting that Cattell, the other great exponent of factor analysis and of a dimensional representation of personality, disagrees sharply with Eysenck on this issue and is emphatic that psychoticism is not normally distributed as a source trait in the general population – 'Most of the abnormality of the neurotic can be expressed as a deviant or unusual pattern in ordinary source traits. . . on the other hand, perhaps half a dozen new factors of an almost purely pathological kind have to be added to a measuring instrument if it is to do justice to the full description of the psychotic' (Cattell, 1970). Recently, Eysenck himself has conceded that in addition to 'the existence of a polygenic factor of psychoticism' there may be 'rather specific genes determining specific expressions of psychoticism, possibly one single gene or small cluster of genes being responsible for manic depressive disorder, another for schizophrenia, and so on' (Verma and Eysenck, 1973). In fact, most of the available genetic evidence is still compatible with multifactorial inheritance for both schizophrenia and manic depressive illness but if specific genes, dominant or recessive, were to be identified, the rationale for a dimensional representation would be irreparably weakened.

*Neurotic illness*

None of these arguments applies with the same force to neurotic illness. Our existing categorical system is highly unreliable and generally regarded as arbitrary and unsatisfactory. So far at least, cluster analysis studies have not revealed stable neurotic clusters and the available evidence suggests that the constitutional basis of neurotic illness is determined by multiple genes of small effect (Miner, 1973). Furthermore, neurotic symptoms are exhibited at times or in mild form by a high proportion of any population that is examined in sufficient detail, and as a result estimates of the prevalence of neurotic symptoms in urban populations have ranged as high as 85 per cent (Srole, Langner, Michael, Opler and Rennie, 1962). The disadvantages of a typology of personality disorder are even more obvious and are well illustrated by a recent study by Presly and Walton (1973). One hundred and forty consecutive admissions to a psychiatric ward, excluding chronic schizophrenics and those with organic illnesses, were allocated to one of eleven categories in a classification of personality types. Although this classification was familiar to all the psychiatrists involved the reliability of their allocations was very low, with disagreements about the type and the severity of the disorder both equally common. The reliability of ratings for the same patients on forty six personality traits, all scored on 4 point scales, was considerably higher, however, and led the authors to conclude that 'a coordinate dimensional approach is to be preferred'. It is worth noting also that the classical German concept of psychopathic personality described so well by Kurt Schneider (1950) is based on an explicitly statistical concept of deviance, and that in listing his ten types, Schneider was at pains to emphasize that he regarded these merely as an unstructured and somewhat idealized list of personality types commonly encountered in psychiatric practice, rather than as discrete entities. Even the classifications devised by Gruhle, Homburger and Kahn at a time when the disease entity was still in its heyday share this dimensional basis, the types they described being regarded in each case as the product of an excess or deficiency of a quality or trait possessed by normal men.

## Statistical considerations

Quite apart from general considerations such as these, there are purely statistical arguments for preferring a dimensional system for neurotic illness and a typology for psychosis. As Maxwell (1972) has shown in an interesting analysis, psychiatrists' ratings of common neurotic symptoms tend to be normally distributed in patient populations with the majority of patients, psychotic and neurotic, scoring at some level in most areas of symptomatology. Data of this sort lend themselves to factor analysis and general factors capable of providing the axes of a dimensional system are readily obtained. Attempts at cluster analysis, on the other hand, tend to be unsuccessful. Ratings of psychotic symptoms have quite a different distribution. Even in psychotic populations most individual symptoms are rare and tend to have a reversed J–shaped distribution with zero scores predominating. Such data are unsuitable for factor analysis and if it is attempted, numerous artefactual factors are obtained, reflecting no more than the presence of small groups of highly correlated symptoms present in a minority of patients. Cluster analysis of such data, however, may well reveal stable clusters. It is, of course, quite possible to omit maldistributed symptoms like hallucinations and delusions and only employ items which are more or less normally distributed. This has often been done, particularly by psychologists, and under these conditions data from psychotic populations can be subjected to factor analysis and genuine dimensions obtained. This is perfectly legitimate provided such data are not used to buttress the argument that there are no qualitative differences between psychosis and normality.

## Conclusions

In spite of the cogent arguments in favour of a dimensional representation of neurotic illness and the similar even stronger arguments relating to personality disorder, there is little evidence that any substantial body of psychiatrists is yet willing to entertain such an innovation. Doubtless this is partly due to a natural conservatism, and apprehension at the prospect of statistical concepts intruding into routine clinical practice, but there are other more substantial reasons also. For many purposes – epidemiological research, the rational planning of medical services and indeed most forms of scientific communication – it is inescapable that patients be divided into groups defined by their common characteristics. The search for clusters of similar individuals standing out against a background of heterogeneity can also be justified even in the absence of good indications that they are likely to be found. This is because a convincing demonstration of clustering is not only an important aid to rational classification but carries aetiological implications of its own. If a group of patients can be found who are strikingly alike in some respect, and different from their fellows, it is likely that this similarity depends on an underlying qualitative difference between them and others, and to identify the cluster accurately is to be half way to identifying this more fundamental difference.

If some of the syndromes we recognize at present, or elements from within them, could be shown to fulfil the 'disease entity' criteria discussed in chapter 5, either by demonstrating the rarity of interforms between them and other adjacent syndromes, or by the discovery of an underlying qualitative abnormality such as a specific gene or biochemical defect, the arguments for a typology would be overwhelming, at least in that area. A dimensional representation would still be possible, but it is difficult to envisage any circumstances in which it would be preferable. If this does not occur, the choice between categories and dimensions will remain more finely balanced. For the forseeable future clinicians are likely to continue to prefer the former for the historical and practical reasons discussed above. Those whose interest is primarily in the nature of the relationship between different syndromes, and between illness and normality, will probably prefer to think in dimensional terms. Nor is there any reason why clinician and theoretician should not differ in this way, particularly now that the dangerous assumptions about the nature of disease inherited from the 19th century have been discarded. In the long run, though, it is difficult to believe that both will not become convinced of the continuity between personality disorders and normal personality, and probably between neurotic illness and normality as well, and hence of the need for a dimensional representation of these phenomena. Whether psychotic illness, or some part of it, will continue to be classified as a number of discrete types or whether it too will come to be represented in dimensional terms only time can tell. It would be rash at this stage to predict, or advocate, either solution with any assurance.

# 10 Defining Diagnostic Criteria

*The vital importance of reproducible criteria*

The various studies described in chapters 3 and 6 make it clear that the reliability of psychiatric diagnosis is often very low, and that diagnostic criteria may vary considerably from one country to another and even between different centres in the same country. Although this situation may not seem very important to busy clinicians intent on treating their patients to the best of their ability, to the research worker it poses great problems, and if the clinician pauses to assess the evidence justifying the therapeutic decisions he makes every day it does the same for him. A glance at a recent issue of any major psychiatric journal makes it clear that the subject matter of most current research is defined, wholly or in part, by diagnostic criteria. Apart from a few studies based explicitly on non-patients and others on populations defined by purely administrative criteria [i.e. all patients admitted to a particular facility between dates A and B] the bulk of contemporary research is based on populations identified and subdivided by diagnostic criteria. But if these criteria are nowhere explicitly stated, are prone to vary from one patient to the next in unpredictable ways, and vary systematically from place to place and time to time, the usefulness of this research is gravely impaired. The findings of any study are only useful to other people if they can be confident, on the basis of the diagnostic and other information provided, that they know what sorts of patients it was based on, and so could, at least in theory, assemble a comparable population themselves and repeat the study.

It is indeed one of the fundamental requirements of all scientific work that it should be carried out and described with sufficient precision for others to be able to repeat it, and this principle applies to the definition of the subject matter just as much as it does to the experimental procedures involved and the results obtained. We have seen that where mental illness is concerned this requirement is met very imperfectly at present. The information that the subjects of a particular study had all been diagnosed as schizophrenics or hysterics often tells us remarkably little about them, certainly not enough for us to be able to assemble another group of patients with any confidence that they would be comparable. It is probably true to say that this failure, or inability, to define adequately the essential common characteristics of the patients who constitute its subject matter, and those of the population from which they were drawn, is the most serious defect of contemporary psychiatric research. The literature is full of studies, highly sophisticated in other respects, with elegant rating techniques and complex statistical handling, which are rendered almost valueless by their neglect of this crucial issue. The purpose of this chapter is to describe some of the ways in which diagnostic criteria could be made more precise without discarding their traditional basis in the patient's symptomatology.

Because the potential unreliability of psychiatric diagnosis is widely recognized, attempts are often made to deal with the problem by ensuring that diagnostic assignments for research purposes are made only by experienced diagnosticians, or that they are agreed by two diagnosticians working independently, or simply by excluding all atypical cases, The literature is full of such phrases as 'diagnosed by Board-certified psychiatrists', 'diagnosed independently by two experienced clinicians', 'all with typical symptoms', 'in no case was there any doubt about the diagnosis', and so on. Unfortunately, although there is probably some value in each of these strategies, they are all hopelessly inadequate. Experienced psychiatrists are perfectly capable of disagreeing with one another, as anyone who has ever attended a case conference will know. Even when two have agreed a third may still fail to do so, and what is regarded as typical schizophrenia in New York may be nothing of the sort in London or Manchester.

For the most part, psychiatric diagnoses are based on symptomatology. Indeed, as Scadding's (1967) lucid analysis of our concept of disease implies, at present the defining characteristic of every non-organic psychiatric diagnosis is simply its syndrome, the constellation of symptoms and signs typically associated with that diagnosis. It is convenient to distinguish two main components to the low reliability of this type of diagnosis: disagreements about which symptoms are present; and disagreements about which symptoms, or combinations of symptoms, are necessary to establish the diagnosis under consideration. It is probably simpler to consider the second of these, the question of diagnostic criteria, first and defer that of symptom detection until later.

DEFINING THE RELATIONSHIP BETWEEN SYMPTOMS AND DIAGNOSIS

The basic problem is that in ordinary clinical practice the relationship between symptoms and diagnosis is inadequately specified. Usually all the characteristic features of any given condition do not have to be present in order to establish that diagnosis. To be diagnosed as a schizophrenic, for instance, a patient does not have to possess all the typical symptoms of schizophrenia, only some of them. But which are essential and which are not, which may be regarded as alternatives to one another, how many must be present altogether, and which other symptoms must be absent, are rarely specified.

Authors sometimes attempt to clarify their diagnostic criteria by stating that they were 'in accordance with the description in Mayer Gross and Slater's (or someone else's) textbook'. Unfortunately such statements are of little value. Textbooks generally provide descriptions of the typical features of syndromes, rather than criteria for establishing their presence, and it is known that psychiatrists may use diagnostic categories in quite different ways in practice, in spite of agreeing on the characteristics possessed by typical members of that category (Hordern, Sandifer, Green and Timbury, 1968).

## The value of glossaries

It has often been suggested that the problem of defining diagnostic criteria could largely be solved by the provision of glossaries containing definitions of all the diagnostic categories recognized in a given nomenclature. It was primarily with this intention that, twenty years ago, the American Psychiatric Association introduced its *Diagnostic and Statistical Manual* (American Psychiatric Association, 1952) and, sixteen years later, that the Registrar General's advisory committee in this country provided a glossary to the Eighth Revision of the *International Classification* (General Register Office, 1968) when that nomenclature was first introduced. In practice, however, both these glossaries have achieved only limited success. This is partly because of the inherent defects of ICD–8, particularly the way in which it chops and changes between symptomatology and aetiology as a basis for classification, but to a large extent it is due to the type of definition provided in these glossaries. As was pointed out in chapter 7, neither really provides adequate working definitions of its various diagnostic categories, much less the true operational definitions advocated by Hempel (1961). For the most part their definitions consist of brief descriptions of the characteristic features of each condition, which provide a useful summary of the essential elements of the clinical concept in question, as ordinary textbook descriptions do, but are of little help in indicating how patients with mixed or atypical symptoms should be classified. For this purpose, a set of clearly defined criteria which *must* be fulfilled, rather than a description of the typical features of the condition, is what is needed. Instead of saying that the typical features of diagnosis X are A,B,C and sometimes D one has to say something like this: To establish diagnosis X, A must be present, together with at least two of the four features B,C,D and E, and P and Q must both be absent. Sets of operational definitions of this type do exist. For example, Feighner, Robins, Guze, Woodruff, Winokur and Munoz (1972) have recently published the criteria used in St Louis for the fifteen major diagnostic categories which they recognize. One may disagree with some of their criteria, or even question some of their categories, but the need for unambiguous criteria of this type can hardly be questioned.

*Descriptive and operational definitions*

The difference between these two types of definition, the descriptive and the operational, is probably best illustrated by example. In the Registrar General's glossary anxiety neurosis is defined as:

'A disorder in which the principal manifestation is excessive anxiety, often amounting to panic, presenting in the psychic and/or somatic field, diffuse in quality, in which other psychoneurotic components such as obsessional or hysterical phenomena, though possibly present, do not dominate the clinical picture.'

By contrast, Feighner and his colleagues give these criteria:

1. 'The following manifestations must be present: (a) Age of onset prior to 40. (b) Chronic nervousness with recurrent anxiety attacks manifested by apprehension, fearfulness, or sense of impending doom, with at least four of the following symptoms present during the majority of attacks: (i) dyspnoea, (ii) palpitations, (iii) chest pain or discomfort (iv) choking or smothering sensation, (v) dizziness and (vi) paraesthesiae.

2. The anxiety attacks are essential to the diagnosis and must occur at times other than marked physical exertion or life-threatening situations, and in the absence of medical illness that *could* account for symptoms of anxiety. There must have been at least six anxiety attacks, each separated by at least a week from the others.

3. In the presence of other psychiatric illness(es) this diagnosis is made *only* if the criteria described in 1 and 2 antedate the onset of the other psychiatric illness by at least two years.'

To know that a group of patients were diagnosed using the Registrar General's criteria is in practice not much more informative than knowing that they were diagnosed 'by experienced psychiatrists', or 'in accordance with the description in so and so's textbook', but to know that the St Louis criteria were used gives a fairly precise indication of which patients would and would not have been included.

*The boundary problem*

In graphical terms a description of the typical clinical features of a diagnostic category identifies its core, the bulls-eye of the target as it were, whereas an operational defininion identifies the boundary between it and other adjacent categories or, to pursue the analogy, the outer rim of the target. It is this boundary or outer rim which matters most. Diagnostic disagreements between psychiatrists, particularly the international differences discussed in chapter 6, are mostly disagreements about the sites of boundaries rather than about the nature of the core symptoms of diagnostic categories. Usually there is agreement on the typical features, and so on typical patients, but one group of psychiatrists has a narrow concept of the condition and insists that these characteristic symptoms be present in full, while another has a much broader concept and only requires some of them to be present. In other words disagreements usually take the form of:

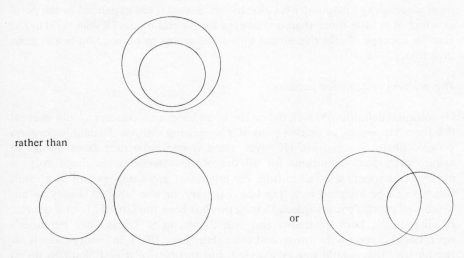

rather than

with the narrower of the two alternative concepts entirely enclosed within its broader competitor.

A second but related reason why it is so important to define the boundary of a category as well as its core is that diagnostic categories seem to possess an innate propensity to expand. Individual clinicians or groups of clinicians with a strong interest in a particular illness almost invariably make that diagnosis more and more readily as time goes on. Usually they regard themselves as having become progressively more skilful at detecting afflicted patients, and doubtless this is sometimes so, but often, like Sir Colenso Ridgeon, all they have really done is to expand the boundaries of their concept of that illness without realizing it. Indeed no very intimate knowledge of the history of psychiatry is required to realize that the natural history of most successful diagnostic concepts is to expand their boundaries ever more and more widely, until eventually they become so overinclusive that they lose all meaning and have to be abandoned. Bumke (1909) described this recurrent phenomenon very well long ago:

'Just as the rings made on the water by raindrops are first small and distinct and then grow larger and larger, swallow each other and vanish, so from time to time in psychiatry there emerge diseases which constantly enlarge themselves until they perish with their own magnitude. Esquirol's monomania, the paranoia of the 'eighties and Meynert's amentia are all examples of this. Hebephrenia and catatonia, which were relatively clearly defined, grew into dementia praecox which seemed to have no limits and folie circulaire into manic-depressive insanity which seemed equally ill-defined.'

The contemporary North American concept of schizophrenia is a classical example of the same phenomenon, and is already heading for the same fate as its predecessors as psychiatrists come to realize that it has expanded to the point at which it is little more than a synonym for mental illness (Kubie, 1971). The English concept of affective illness sometimes seems to be heading in the same direction.

### The problem of excluded patients

Operational definitions which define the boundaries of a concept would prevent this from happening, or at least prevent it happening without the defining criteria being deliberately changed. However, there is one important disadvantage to using operational definitions for all diagnostic categories simultaneously: a number of patients will fail to fulfil the criteria of any category and as a result will have to be assigned to a 'rag bag' category, or else labelled simply as 'un-diagnosed psychiatric disorder'. In fact, this has been the fate of about a quarter of all patients, both inpatients and outpatients, in St Louis since Feighner's operational criteria were introduced there (Hudgens, 1971). In theory there is no reason why this should not be avoided, but in practice it is difficult to do so without either making the classification so simple that it fails to represent the clinical concepts it is concerned with, or alternatively making the diagnostic criteria for each condition so complex and interdependent that they can barely be understood. Part of the problem is that ordinary language is not an appropriate medium for expressing the complex rules needed to cope with innumerable combinations of symptoms. The notation of symbolic logic (Ledley and Lusted, 1959) is really required in this situation, but any glossary couched in these terms would be quite unsuitable for ordinary clinical use.

### Choosing appropriate criteria

In some kinds of research, particularly biological studies, it is vital to ensure that all those who are included are correctly diagnosed but immaterial how many others are excluded or left undiagnosed in the process. In a situation like this there are a number of acceptable ways in which the diagnostic composition of the subject matter could be defined. A publicly available set of operational criteria, of the type described by Feighner and his colleagues, could be used for each diagnostic category involved. In many ways this is the ideal solution as there are obvious advantages in a single set of criteria becoming widely accepted and used in many different centres. But often no suitable criteria are available and the researcher has to produce a working definition of his own which corresponds reasonably well to the clinical concept in question and at the same time stipulates exactly which patients should and should not be included. For instance, manic depressive depression could be defined as severe depression of mood in the presence of any two of the following; severe weight loss, early morning wakening, guilt feelings, diurnal variation of mood, retardation and a 'distinct quality' to the depression. Or schizophrenia could be defined as an illness characterized by the presence of any one of Schneider's 'symptoms of the first rank' (Mellor, 1970) in the absence of evidence of brain disease. If suitable rating scales exist it is usually preferable to frame the definition in terms of scores on these, because in this way relatively complex criteria, involving numerous alternative combinations of symptoms, can be expressed quite simply without any loss of clarity. Manic depressive depression, for instance, might be defined by a score of 8 or more on the Newcastle Scale (Carney, Roth and Garside, 1965), or schizophrenia as a score of 4 or more on the New Haven Schizophrenia Index (Astrachan, Harrow, Adler, Brauer, Schwartz and Tucker, 1972).

If only a small number of patients are needed, but it is important for them to be classical cases, criteria of this sort can easily be made more stringent. For a diagnosis of schizophrenia, two first rank symptoms could be required instead of one, for manic depressive illness a score of 10 on the Newcastle Scale might be required instead of 8, and so on. In practice where the line is drawn will depend on how many patients are needed and how much time is available. In a drug trial, for instance, criteria that were too restrictive might jeopardize the chances of the trial ever being completed. What matters is that there should be clear and uniform criteria for each diagnostic category. What those criteria are and how restrictive they are are subsidiary issues.

Situations in which it is necessary for every subject in a population to be allocated to a diagnostic category, as is the case in epidemiological studies, are much harder to deal with. As no one can be rejected or left undiagnosed, rules of class membership must be laid down within a unitary framework and as a result they usually become very complex. If the number of symptoms recognized and the number of diagnostic categories involved are both fairly small these rules can be instituted by hand, as in Silbermann's CHAM system (1971), but it is generally necessary, for reasons of both speed and accuracy, to utilize a computer and most existing systems do so.

*Diagnosis by computer*

Three quite different types of computer program have been used for this purpose; those based on a logical decision tree, those based on probability theory, and those based on discriminant function procedures. All three are described in more detail in the next chapter, so only a few general comments are appropriate here. A logical decision tree has the same formal structure as that of the flora most of us used at school to identify flowers from the shape and number of their leaves, petals, stamens etc. It consists simply of a series of questions, the answer to each of which eliminates one or more diagnoses or groups of diagnoses and also determines the next question asked, until eventually every diagnosis but one has been eliminated. What that diagnosis is depends on the arbitrary rules of which the decision tree is composed. The skill in designing a program of this kind lies in producing a set of rules that will produce diagnoses that experienced clinicians would consider appropriate.

The other two approaches, one based on probability theory (Bayes' Theorem) and the other on discriminant functions, both involve complicated statistical procedures, and assumptions, but have the advantage that the diagnoses they generate can be accompanied by an estimate of the likelihood of their being correct, and also by alternative diagnoses if need be. However, the Bayesian model involves knowing beforehand, or being able to produce a reasonable estimate of, the incidence of each symptom in each of the diagnoses under consideration; and discriminant functions have to be generated in the first place from data from a large series of patients, each supplied with a clinical diagnosis and rated for the presence or absence of all the N symptoms from which the various diagnostic distinctions involved are derived.

All three methods ensure that the same combination of symptoms will always generate the same diagnosis and, in the context with which we are concerned, this is their importance. Although different programs may produce different diagnoses from the same symptoms, any individual program will always be consistent, regardless of what its own internal statistical or logical basis may be.

SYMPTOM DETECTION

So far we have been concerned entirely with various ways of ensuring that any given combination of symptoms always leads to the same diagnosis, without considering how the presence of those symptoms is established in the first place. Unfortunately disagreements about symptomatology are just as common as those about diagnosis, and even harder to eliminate.

*Traditional methods*

Traditionally psychiatrists, like other physicians, have detected symptoms by holding a free-ranging interview with the patient, and perhaps with his relatives also, and have been accustomed to assume that the symptoms they elicited were present and that those they did not elicit were absent. Unfortunately, these happy assumptions are unwarranted, as the first reliability studies soon revealed. To quote but one example, when pairs of experienced psychiatrists interviewed a series of ninety outpatients independently within a few days of one another and recorded the presence or absence of twenty four clinical items in each, the average positive percentage agreement was only 46 per cent. In other words, when one psychiatrist recorded a symptom as present there was less than a 50–50 chance of his colleague agreeing with him. (Kreitman, Sainsbury, Morrissey, Towers and Scrivener, 1961.)

Many factors contribute to this low reliability. There are differences in behaviour between one psychiatrist and another; they ask different questions, show interest and probe further in different places, establish different sorts of relationship with the patient, and so on. Then there are differences in expectation, which tend in a variety of ways to facilitate the detection of what is expected and militate against the detection or recognition of the unexpected to a quite surprising extent (Kendell, 1968b). Finally, important conceptual differences are often involved. Common technical terms like anxiety, delusion, thought disorder and so on may be used in quite different ways by different psychiatrists without their being aware that this is so (see Rosenzwieg, Vandenberg, Moore and Dukay, 1961); and even where there is no disagreement over the meaning of a term there is often disagreement over the extent to which graded characteristics like worry or tension have to be present to justify a positive rating.

TABLE 3 The main sources of unreliability in the clinical interview, and the effect on these of Questionnaires, Rating Scales and Structured Interviews.

| Source of Unreliability | Self-Assessment Questionnaire | Rating Scale | Structured Interview |
|---|---|---|---|
| The Interviewer's behaviour | Eliminated | May be limited to some extent | Severely limited by procedural rules |
| The Interviewer's expectations | Eliminated | Largely unaffected | Limited by procedural rules |
| The Interviewer's interpretation of the technical terms involved. | Problem transferred to the patient. | Can be reduced by providing definitions. | Reduced by the provision of definitions. |

A growing awareness of these problems has led to the development of three fairly distinct groups of instruments – self-assessment questionnaires, rating scales and structured interviews. They avoid or minimize the short-comings of the traditional clinical interview in different ways and to differing extents (see Table 3) and each has important advantages and disadvantages.

*Self-assessment questionnaires*

These eliminate the interview completely. In this way they remove at one stroke all the problems produced by the vagaries of the clinician, but in doing so create several others instead. Patients who are agitated, retarded, unable to concentrate, or badly disturbed in any way, may give very misleading answers. It is comparatively easy for symptoms to be denied; patients' actual behaviour, as opposed to their views about it, cannot be examined at all; and there is no more guarantee that different patients all mean the same by words like anxious, depressed and hostile than there is that different interviewers do so. For these reasons, questionnaires are usually inappropriate in situations where it is necessary to establish accurately the presence or absence of particular symptoms in individual patients. In general they are most useful for measuring overall levels of pathology in populations which do not contain a high proportion of disturbed or psychotic people, for measuring change in particular aspects of psychopathology like depression or anxiety, and as screening devices for the detection of psychiatric disturbance. In fact, the majority of widely used questionnaires were specially designed for one of these three purposes. The Beck Inventory (Beck, Ward, Mendelson, Mock and Erbaugh, 1961) and the Zung Self Rating Depressive Scale (Zung, 1965) were designed specifically to measure change in depressive symptomatology over time and the Taylor Manifest Anxiety Scale (Taylor, 1953) was designed to fulfil an analogous function for symptoms of anxiety. Goldberg's General Health Questionnaire (Goldberg, 1972) was developed specifically to detect patients with significant psychiatric problems in general medical populations and Hathaway and McKinley's Minnesota Multiphasic Personality Inventory (MMPI), though originally introduced as a screening instrument for military recruits, has since been used most successfully for comparing overall levels or patterns of symptomatology in different populations.

*Rating scales*

Rating scales provide a convenient means of ensuring that a predetermined range of topics will be covered in a clinical interview and that the information elicited in these areas will be recorded in a uniform way. They hold strong attractions for statistically minded researchers because they ensure that the data arrive in a form suitable for whatever statistical manipulations are envisaged and, because they are so easy to construct, they are often designed on an ad hoc basis for individual pieces of research. If adequate working definitions are provided for the various items of psychopathology contributing to the scale reliability may be quite high, in spite of the fact that the interviewer is left to elicit the necessary information however he likes. If this is not done, however, a rating scale is simply an unstructured clinical interview covering a particular range of topics and retains all the shortcomings of an ordinary interview beneath its veneer of respectability. Lorr's In-Patient Multidimensional Psychiatric Scale (Lorr and Klett, 1967) and Overall's Brief Psychiatric Rating Scale (Overall and Gorham, 1962) have both been widely used and cover the range of psychopathology likely to be elicited in a clinical interview. Lorr's IMPS contains eighty nine items, mostly rated on 9 point scales, and the need for definitions is circumvented fairly successfully by a careful avoidance of all technical terms. The first question, for instance, asks not whether the patient is verbally retarded but whether, 'compared to the normal person' his speech is 'slowed, deliberate or laboured'. Overall's BPRS consists of sixteen 7 point scales embracing different areas of symtomatology and reasonably adequate working definitions are provided for each of them. The main use of both these instruments is for comparing levels and patterns of symptomatology in different populations, English and West Indian schizophrenics for example, or for measuring change in a single population, as in drug trials. Like self-rating questionnaires, they are not usually suitable in situations in which it is crucial, for diagnostic or other reasons, to establish the presence or absence of individual items of psychopathology.

*Structured interviews*

Structured or standardized interviews are of more recent origin than questionnaires or rating scales and to some extent their development is the result of an increasing recognition of the inadequacies of these other instruments. In a structured interview the manner in which symptoms are elicited is prescribed as well as the way in which they are recorded. The questions the patient is asked, and their order, are both laid down in advance, ratings are made serially as the interview progresses rather than at the end, and definitions, implicit or explicit, are provided for each item. Actually the degree of standardization involved varies considerably. In some instruments, as in Burdock's Structured Clinical Interview (Burdock and Hardesty, 1969), what the interviewer can say and do is so tightly controlled that it is very close to being a verbally administered questionnaire. In others the interviewer still retains some control over the exact wording of the questions he asks and even over his interpretation of the patient's replies.

The differences between these two approaches are exemplified by the two most well known and widely used structured interviews, Spitzer's Psychiatric Status Schedule (Spitzer, Endicott, Fleiss and Cohen, 1970) and Wing's Present State Examination (Wing, Cooper and Sartorius, 1974). The Psychiatric Status Schedule (PSS) is designed to elicit and record the symptoms experienced by the patient and his role functioning during the preceding 7 days and consists of a booklet containing an interview schedule and a matching inventory of 321 dichotomous items. The schedule stipulates the exact form of words to be used for each question and the corresponding ratings are closely tied to the wording of the patient's reply. Further probing is allowed if his reply is incomplete or ambiguous, but only to a limited extent, by means of general queries like 'Can you tell me more about that?' or 'What do you mean by that?' The Present State Examination (PSE) is less highly structured and also differs in other ways. It is concerned more exclusively with symptoms, particularly psychotic phenomena, and covers a longer period of time, the previous 4 weeks rather than the previous 7 days. Suggested probes are provided for each item but with this instrument the interviewer is free to ask additional questions if he considers it necessary, and the rating he finally makes represents *his* judgement whether or not the symptom in question is present, rather than the patient's initial reply to his original probe.

In theory the PSS, as the more highly structured of the two, should have higher reliability. In practice, it is possible to obtain equally good reliability with the PSE, though only after prolonged training. Both interviews can be used comfortably with a wide range of patients and are equipped with decision tree computer programs (Diagno and Catego – see chapter 11) to convert symptom profiles into diagnoses. The PSS requires less training, can be used by non-psychiatrists, and is perhaps most suitable for population comparisons. The PSE can only really be used by trained psychiatrists, but its flexibility makes it particularly suitable for use with psychotic patients or in situations where the patient's symptoms need to be elicited in detail. Several other structured interviews have been developed, including history interviews. Indeed, Spitzer and his colleagues have produced a veritable arsenal of instruments for use in different situations (Spitzer, Endicott and Fleiss, 1967).

Their relative lack of flexibility, and the training needed to use them fluently and reliably, makes structured interviews inappropriate for ordinary clinical purposes. They are essentially research instruments. Whether they should be regarded as essential in any given piece of clinical research depends on the circumstances. In cross-cultural comparisons where it is vital for geographically separated groups of patients to be interviewed in identical ways, or in any multi-centre study involving more than one team of interviewers, they are obviously essential. In a situation where only a small group of interviewers and one patient population are involved the need is less obvious, particularly as in situations of this sort it is often possible to demonstrate adequate reliability using a rating scale. Even here though, the general requirement of all scientific work, that what is done should be stipulated and described with sufficient precision for others to be able to do the same, makes it difficult to defend unstructured interviewing, especially if operational definitions are not provided for all the technical terms involved.

*Semantic and syntactical definitions*

The crucial role of adequate definitions is a constant theme running through this discussion. Indeed it is the dominant theme of this whole book. They are as important for symptoms or individual items of psychopathology as they are for diagnoses and it is much easier to provide them for some symptoms than for others. Weight loss can easily be defined as 'loss of at least 3 kg in 6 months in the absence of relevant organic disease or deliberate dieting' and early morning wakening as 'waking, and failing to return to sleep, at least 2 hours before normal at least 3 nights a week'. Items like 'good previous personality' and 'immaturity' pose a much harder problem. It is relatively easy to provide terms such as these with 'syntactical' definitions which provide rules of substitution, but much harder to provide 'semantic' definitions providing rules of application (Reid and Finesinger, 1952). For example, it is relatively easy to define immaturity as 'failure to develop the attitudes and behaviour patterns generally accepted as appropriate to the individual's chronological age', but syntactical definitions like this do not make it any clearer which people the term is applicable to. All they really do is provide an alternative form of words allowing us, if we wish, to avoid using the word 'immaturity'. A semantic definition, on the other hand, would have to specify precisely which attitudes and behaviours were evidence of immaturity and which were not, and in practice this is very difficult to do. For this reason terms like 'immaturity' and 'good previous personality' are best avoided. In general, all definitions which remain heavily dependent on inference, as purely syntactical definitions inevitably do, are likely to prove inadequate, as there is abundant evidence that inferential judgements are consistently less reliable than those based on directly observable criteria (Heyns and Lippitt, 1954; Lehmann, Ban and Donald, 1965). In principle there is no reason why patients should not be classified on the basis of the defence mechanisms they utilize rather than their overt symptoms, particularly as many psychiatrists believe that such a classification would be more useful and valuable than our present one. The problem is that the majority of the psychoanalytic concepts involved cannot be provided with semantic or operational definitions, or at least their advocates are not prepared to reformulate them in such a way as to make this possible. As a result, the reliability of these terms remains so low that any attempt to use them as a basis for classification is hamstrung from the start.

*The value of physiological and psychological tests*

Sometimes it is possible to use physiological or psychological test results as defining criteria, though usually only as an adjunct to clinical criteria. For instance, a minimum level of 'basal' forearm blood flow of 4 ml/100 ml/min (Kelly, 1966) might be used as a qualifying condition in a study of anxiety states, or a stipulated range of intensity and consistency scores on the Bannister Fransella Grid Test as a qualifying condition in a study of thought-disordered schizophrenics (Bannister and Fransella, 1966). In general, opportunities of this sort should always be taken as physiological or psychological tests are likely to be more reliable than purely clinical criteria, if only because they do not depend on subjective or inferential judgements. However, it is important to establish the reliability of a test in the circumstances in which it is to be used before deciding to use it. A test that has been shown to be reliable when administered by its originator to student volunteers will not necessarily be reliable when administered by others to chronic schizophrenics. Validity must also be considered. In some circumstances a clinical rating of anxiety may be preferable to physiological measures like palmar skin conductance or forearm electromyography in spite of its comparatively low reliability because it is a direct measure of the variable in question, the subjective experience of anxiety, whereas the others are only indirectly related to this.

CONCLUSIONS

There is a common theme to the various measures that have been advocated in this chapter, and the various techniques and instruments that have been described. All of them are concerned with tightening up the relationship either between the patient's complaints and behaviour and the symptoms attributed to him, or between these symptoms and the diagnosis derived from them. Some, like the use of computer programs for producing diagnoses from symptom patterns, require facilities which at present are only available in a few centres, others may only be necessary in particular circumstances. However, all of them are means of tackling the central issue of definition. Directly or indirectly they are all ways of providing the technical terms we use to describe the phenomena of mental illness with adequate 'semantic' or 'operational' definitions. Provided this is done somehow, the precise means employed is of secondary importance. And if every term is adequately defined properly trained raters will be able to achieve acceptable levels of reliability, and the unrecognized differences in usage between one centre and another that have plagued us in the past can be expected to fade away.

# 11 Diagnosis by Computer

The development in recent years of computer programs for generating diagnoses from symptom patterns was referred to briefly in the previous chapter. The reasons why these programs have been produced have also been discussed previously. Their main attraction is that, whatever their logical or statistical basis, all computer programs are completely reliable. Any given combination of symptoms or clinical ratings will invariably generate the same diagnosis every time, thereby completely eliminating one of the main sources of the low reliability and geographical instability of diagnoses made by clinicians. Although similar programs have been developed to replace or augment clinical diagnosis in other branches of medicine, their potential value is particularly clear where mental illness is concerned. This is partly because the low reliability and variable usage which result from employing imprecise diagnostic criteria tend to be more of a problem in psychiatry than elsewhere, and partly because the effective utilization of computer programs in other areas is hampered by the variable conceptual basis of different illnesses. As Scadding (1967) has pointed out, if one condition is defined on the basis of its morbid anatomy, another on the basis of a physiological disturbance and a third on the basis of a biochemical or chromosomal anomaly, as is the case in many branches of medicine, it is extremely difficult to allocate diagnoses within the sort of unitary framework which a computer requires without misrepresenting the defining characteristics of some of them. This problem does not arise where psychiatry is concerned because nearly all mental illnesses are still defined in clinical-descriptive terms. This homogeneous conceptual basis, which in other settings is rightly regarded as evidence of the backwardness of psychiatry, is actually an asset in this particular situation.

## The advantages of computer programs

The increased reliability and stability of diagnoses generated by a computer produces obvious benefits in the context either of a research study or of the administration and planning of clinical services. These benefits have been discussed before and there is no need to repeat the argument here. If the quality of the data which constitute the program's input is low the gain may be fairly slight, but diagnoses derived by a computer from unreliable data will still be at least as useful as those derived from the same data by other means. But the development and progressive refinement of computer programs for generating diagnoses have other less immediate but equally important consequences. By creating, as they do, a range of experimental models simulating the process by which clinicians arrive at diagnoses, they focus attention on the largely unexplored mechanisms of diagnostic pattern recognition and decision making. By producing, as they also do, a variety of alternative diagnostic criteria, each of them explicit and available for public scrutiny, they serve to focus attention on the neglected issue of the validity of our diagnoses. Consider, for example, a situation in which three different programs are in use simultaneously, all embodying different concepts of schizophrenia. In such a situation psychiatrists would be forced to consider which of the three concepts was the most useful, and in so doing to decide what their criterion of usefulness or validity was to be. Alternatively, a situation might well arise in which one particular program came into general use, perhaps in combination with a particular interviewing schedule or rating scale. Such a development would have profound implications, much greater than those accompanying the popularization of other instruments like the MMPI or the Rorschach Test. For whoever exports his program also exports his diagnostic criteria. We could well find that the diagnostic criteria currently used in one particular country, or even in a particular university department, might come into general use in the wake of the widespread adoption of a popular computer program embodying those criteria. For these and other reasons the application of computer technology to psychiatric diagnosis may prove to be a development of much greater moment than is yet apparent.

DECISION TREE PROGRAMS

Three quite different kinds of computer program have been used for generating diagnoses; those based on a logical decision tree, those based on probability theory and those based on multiple discriminant functions. The decision tree method is the easiest to understand for those with little knowledge of statistics for the simple reason that it does not involve any. It consists purely of a series of questions each of which has to be answered yes or no. Each successive answer eliminates one or more diagnoses or groups of diagnoses and also determines the next question asked, until every diagnosis but one has been eliminated. For example, the first question, based on a group of items concerned with cognitive functioning, might be used to determine whether the illness was organic or not. If the answer was 'no' the second question, based perhaps on a series of items about delusions and hallucinations, might determine whether the illness was psychotic or neurotic, and so on. In this way every possible combination of symptoms is reduced to one or other of the diagnoses recognized in the system. Individual questions may specify the presence of a single item, or that a score derived from several items should lie within a certain range, or be based on complex alternatives involving numerous items in different combinations. The formal structure of a decision tree is actually the same as that of a railway marshalling yard, with patients corresponding to individual trucks, the yes/no questions to sets of points and the trains at the bottom of the yard to diagnoses. When it starts its journey at the top of the yard each truck has the potential to join any of the trains, but each time it passes a set of points its choice becomes more restricted until eventually it is committed to one particular train.

## Diagno

Spitzer's Diagno (Spitzer and Endicott, 1968) was the first program of this type to be developed. It is based on the thirty nine scale scores of a structured mental state interview known as the Psychiatric Status Schedule (see chapter 10) and allocates every patient to one of twenty seven diagnostic categories, including 'not ill' and 'non-specific illness with mild symptomatology'. It was soon followed by Diagno II (Spitzer and Endicott, 1969), a more complex program containing fifty seven decision points compared with Diagno's thirty six and incorporating a limited capacity to revise decisions made at an earlier stage in the sequence. This program utilizes historical data in addition to mental state information in the form of the Current and Past Psychopathology Scales (CAPPS – see Endicott and Spitzer, 1972) and generates a total of forty six different diagnoses, including personality disorders. In a study based on 100 sets of CAPPS ratings, and using $K_w$ as an index of concordance. Spitzer and Endicott were able to show that the diagnostic agreement between Diagno II and clinicians was as good as that between one clinician and another, thus demonstrating the face validity as well as the reliability of the computer's diagnoses.

## Catego

More recently Wing and his colleagues (Wing, Cooper and Sartorius, 1974) have developed a similar program, known as Catego, based on their structured Present State Examination. The design of this program is rather different from that of Diagno. Instead of single diagnoses or groups of diagnoses being eliminated one by one the original input, which consists of 350 PSE items, passes through a progressive series of condensations and all decisions about actual diagnoses are postponed until the final stage. The 350 items are first reduced to 140 'symptoms' and these in turn reduced to thirty five 'syndromes'. Next these syndromes are

11

condensed to six 'descriptive categories'. Up to this stage there is no restriction on the number of elements which any individual patient may exhibit but in the next stage, whether the patient has previously qualified for one descriptive category or all six, his symptomatology is reduced to a single 'descriptive class'. Essentially the same procedure is carried out independently with other data (if it is available) for all previous episodes of illness and the final 'provisional diagnostic class' is then derived from the separate descriptive class assignments of all episodes of illness, past or present. The Catego program prints out all the symptoms, syndromes and descriptive categories exhibited by each individual patient, together with a rough three point ranking ( ?, +, and + +) for each, in addition to the final 'provisional diagnostic class' or diagnosis. In this way much useful information is provided in a standardized form which enables unusual or borderline patients to be distinguished from those with typical symptom patterns.

The potential of this and similar programs was well illustrated in the International Pilot Study of Schizophrenia where it was used to derive standard 'diagnoses' from the PSE ratings of all 1200 patients from the nine countries involved (WHO, 1973a). In this way, several important similarities and differences in the range of patient types encountered in the nine countries were exposed, and also important similarities and differences in the diagnostic criteria of the local psychiatrists in each centre.

PROBABILISTIC METHODS

The second approach is a probabilistic or statistical one based on Bayes' theorem. The basic statement of this theorem is:

$$P(d_i/s_j) = \frac{P(d_i) \cdot P(s_j/d_i)}{\sum P(d_k) \cdot P(s_i/d_k)}$$

where

$P(d_i/s_j)$    is the probability that a patient with the constellation of symptoms $s_j$ has the disease $d_i$.

$P(d_i)$    is the probability (or incidence) of the disease $d_i$ in the population under consideration.

$P(s_j/d_i)$    is the incidence of the symptoms $s_j$ in the disease $d_i$.

$P(d_k)$    is the incidence of each disease $1 \rightarrow k$ in the population.

and

$P(s_j/d_k)$    is the incidence of the symptoms $s_j$ in each of the diseases $1 \rightarrow k$.

Most of the early programs for deriving psychiatric diagnoses by computer were of this type (Birnbaum and Maxwell, 1961; Overall and Gorham, 1963; Overall and Hollister, 1964; Smith, 1966) but, in spite of the obvious relevance of probability theory to diagnosis, the Bayesian model has several disadvantages. It assumes that each of the symptoms $1 \rightarrow j$ is independent of the others and that the diseases $1 \rightarrow k$ are similarly independent of one another. In fact, neither of these assumptions is justified, though symptom independence can be artificially produced by replacing the actual ratings by principal components derived from them. The Bayesian model also requires a reasonable estimate of the incidence of the various symptoms $1 \rightarrow j$ in each of the diseases $1 \rightarrow k$ in the population under consideration, and a similar estimate of the relative frequency of these diseases in that population. In practice these data are rarely available and both Overall and Smith were forced to resort to the questionable procedure of using ratings of hypothetical typical cases to provide their estimates of the distributions of symptoms across diseases, and also to assume that each disease was equally probable.

DISCRIMINANT FUNCTIONS

The third group of techniques is based on the discriminant function procedures introduced by Fisher (1936) and Rao (1948). They are described in more detail in chapter 8, but in its simplest form discriminant analysis involves two populations, one whose members have been assigned a clinical diagnosis A and the other a diagnosis B, and all of whom have been rated for the presence or absence of N items relevant to the distinction between A and B. Starting with these data the anlaysis produces a linear variable (the discriminant function) consisting of a set of weights for the N items calculated so as to maximize the ratio of between-group to within-group variance. As a result, when a score is derived for each patient by adding together his weighted scores on the N items, the separation between those with diagnosis A and those with diagnosis B is maximal. Subsequently, this discriminant function can be used to allocate any patient who has been rated on the N items to the appropriate diagnosis, A or B. In practice several diagnoses are usually involved, not just two, which means using a multiple stepwise discriminant procedure, but the basic principle remains unchanged. Techniques of this sort have been used by Melrose, Stroebel and Glueck (1970) in Connecticut and Sletten, Ulett, Altman and Sunderland (1970) in Missouri. The latter at least were able to obtain a level of agreement between clinical and computer diagnoses comparable to that achieved by Spitzer with Diagno II and have since developed this computer service as a routine procedure in all the psychiatric hospitals in the Missouri State system (Sletten, Altman and Ulett, 1971). Using data from a mental state examination and standard demographic information the central computer provides for each patient within minutes, or at most a few hours, the probabilities of that patient belonging to each of eight broad diagnostic groupings [acute organic brain syndrome, paranoid schizophrenia, personality disorder, etc.]

*The relative merits of the three approaches*

It is debatable which of these three approaches corresponds most closely to the reasoning processes employed by clinicians. Claims have been made on behalf of all three, each of them with some justification. Really we know too little about the decision-making processes of clinicians to decide, and it may well be that they use different strategies in different situations. The hierarchical nature of most of our classifications, with each diagnosis excluding the presence of those that precede it and encompassing the symptoms of those that follow it, strongly suggests a sequence of decisions akin to that of a decision tree. On the other hand, clinicians are clearly influenced by considerations of relative probability comparable to those embodied in Bayes' Theorem. And when concerned with a particular differential diagnosis they may well allocate rough weights to the symptoms suggesting each of the two diagnoses and compare them in much the same way as a simple discriminant procedure does.

It is also arguable which of the three is the most useful. The decision tree method is the simplest, and also the easiest to construct, but each program is usable only with the particular rating scale or structured interview for which it was designed and individual diagnostic distinctions are necessarily based on rather crude criteria. The two statistical procedures share the important advantage that they provide not just a single diagnosis but an estimate, expressed as a probability by the Bayes method and as a distance by the discriminant function method, of how closely the patient resembles typical members of several different categories, thus allowing meaningful alternative diagnoses to be provided and distinguishing typical cases from those with unusual or borderline symptoms. However, both have disadvantages also. As we have already seen, Bayes' theorem makes the unjustified assumption that both symptoms and diagnoses are independent of one another, and also requires prior knowledge of the distributions of symptoms across diseases and, to achieve its full potential, prior knowledge of the relative incidence of the diseases under consideration as well. Discriminant function procedures start with several advantages. They involve fewer unfulfilled assumptions than the probabilistic approach, can handle numeric data without having to break them up into arbitrary nominal groups as the other two methods do, and have the ability to focus large amounts of data onto individual diagnostic discriminations to optimum effect. Their big disadvantage is that the linear functions they utilize have to be derived in the first place from ratings on large populations of patients, the size of the requisite population being governed by the product of the number of separate ratings or scores being used and the number of diagnostic categories to be distinguished. In practice, this means that unless a thousand or more sets of ratings are available one either has to confine oneself to distinguishing a small number of broad diagnostic groups, or make unjustified assumptions about variances and correlations across diagnostic categories and so fail to achieve anything like maximal discrimination. A second problem common to both the statistical methods is that, because their ground rules are derived in the first place from clinical ratings and diagnoses, the short-comings of these data are incorporated into the resulting program. If the initial data are unreliable and biased the program's rules will necessarily be in some respects inappropriate, and its discriminating power blunted as a result. This has two important consequences. The failure of a Bayesian or discriminant function program to generate appropriate diagnoses may be due to the short-comings of the clincial data from which it was derived rather than to the inherent short-comings of the statistical method. Conversely an improvement in the quality of the original developmental data may be expected to result in improved performance by the program.

Fleiss and his colleagues (Fleiss, Spitzer, Cohen and Endicott, 1972) have recently compared the efficacy of a logical decision tree program (Diagno II), a Bayesian program and a multiple discriminant function procedure at distinguishing twelve broad diagnostic categories in a series of 740 patients rated on the CAPPS. Over half these patients had to be used for developing the statistical rules of the Bayesian and discriminant function programs and the actual comparison was therefore restricted to the remaining 286 patients. Using $K_w$ as an index of the degree of concordance between the original clinical diagnoses and the corresponding computer categories they found little difference between the three approaches; $K_w$ lay between 0·43 and 0·48 for all three. However, the discriminant function program was less successful than the other two in reproducing the percentage distribution of the clinicians' diagnoses, mainly because it overdiagnosed paranoid schizophrenia at the expense of non-paranoid forms. When a second comparison was carried out on quite different data – CAPPS ratings obtained from a series of 435 women from an obstetric ward, and so with a much lower overall psychiatric morbidity than the previous material – Diagno came out best with an average $K_w$ for concordance with the clinicians' diagnoses of 0·36, compared with 0·28 for the discriminant function program, and 0·20 for the Bayesian approach. The authors concluded from these results that 'at the present time, a logical decision tree method such as Diagno II is preferable for computer diagnosis to the Bayes and discriminant function methods'. This is a fair assessment of the current situation, though it is likely that discriminant function procedures will eventually prove superior once the practical problems of obtaining sufficiently large series of patients for developmental purposes have been overcome. The appropriate choice in any given situation will also be influenced by other considerations peculiar to that situation – how valuable it would be to have alternative diagnoses available as well as a single 'first choice' diagnosis, whether a wide range of separate diagnoses are needed or only an accurate assignment to a few major categories, and whether or not sufficient data are available to provide an adequate developmental sample for either of the statistical methods.

# References

ALBEE, G. W. (1970). Notes towards a position paper opposing psychodiagnosis. *In New Approaches to Personality Classification*, ed. Mahrer, A. R. pp. 385–395. New York: Columbia University Press.

AMERICAN PSYCHIATRIC ASSOCIATION. (1952) *Diagnostic and Statistical Manual of Mental Disorders*, 1st edn. (DSM–I), Washington, DC: APA.

AMERICAN PSYCHIATRIC ASSOCIATION. (1968) *Diagnostic and Statistical Manual of Mental Disorders*, 2nd edn. (DSM–II), Washington, DC: APA.

ARMITAGE, P. (1971) *Statistical Methods in Medical Research*. p. 336. Oxford: Blackwell Scientific Publications.

ASH, P. (1949) The reliability of psychiatric diagnoses, *Journal of Abnormal and Social Psychology*, **44,** 272–276.

ASTRACHAN, B. M., HARROW, M., ADLER, D., BRAUER, L., SCHWARTZ, C. & TUCKER, G. (1972) A checklist for the diagnosis of schizophrenia, *British Journal of Psychiatry*, **121,** 529–539.

ASTRUP, C. & ∅DEGAARD, ∅. (1970) Continued experiments in psychiatric diagnosis. *Acta Psychiatrica Scandinavica*, **46,** 180–209.

BANNISTER, D. & FRANSELLA, F. (1966) A grid test of schizophrenic thought disorder. *British Journal of Social and Clinical Psychology*, **5,** 95–102.

BANNISTER, D., SALMON, P. & LEIBERMAN, D. M. (1964) Diagnosis-treatment relationships in psychiatry: a statistical analysis. *British Journal of Psychiatry*, **110,** 726–732.

BECK, A. T. (1962) Reliability of psychiatric diagnoses: a critique of systematic studies. *American Journal of Psychiatry*, **119,** 210–216.

BECK, A. T., WARD, C., MENDELSON, M., MOCK, J. & ERBAUGH, J. (1961) An inventory for measuring depression. *Archives of General Psychiatry*, **4,** 561–571.

BECK, A. T., WARD, C., MENDELSON, M., MOCK, J. & ERBAUGH, J. (1962) Reliability of psychiatric diagnoses: 2. A study of consistency of clinical judgements and ratings. *American Journal of Psychiatry*, **119,** 351–357.

BIRNBAUM, A. & MAXWELL, A. E. (1961) Classification procedures based on Bayes' formula. *Applied Statistics*, **9,** 152–169.

BOISEN, A. T. (1938) Types of dementia praecox: a study in psychiatric classification. *Psychiatry*, **1,** 233–236.

BRIDGMAN, P. W. (1927) *The Logic of Modern Physics*, New York: Macmillan.

BUMKE, O. (1909) Über die Umgrenzung des manisch-depressiven Irreseins. *Zentralblatt für Nervenheilkunde und Psychiatrie*, **20,** 381–403.

BURDOCK, E. I. & HARDESTY, A. S. (1969) *Structured Clinical Interview Manual*, New York: Springer.

CAMERON, D. E. (1953) A theory of diagnosis. In *Current Problems in Psychiatric Diagnosis*, eds. Hoch, P. H. & Zubin, J., pp. 33–45. New York: Grune and Stratton.

CARNEY, M. W. P., ROTH, M. & GARSIDE, R. F. (1965) The diagnosis of depressive syndromes and the prediction of E.C.T. response. *British Journal of Psychiatry*, **111,** 659–674.

CATTELL, R. B. (1970) The integration of functional and psychometric requirements in a quantitative and computerised diagnostic system. In *New Approaches to Personality Classification*, ed. Mahrer, A. R. pp. 9–52. New York: Columbia University Press.

CLAUSEN, J. A. (1971) Psychosocial diagnosis: what and why? *American Journal of Orthopsychiatry*, **41**, 847–848.

COHEN, H. (1943) *The Nature, Method and Purpose of Diagnosis*, Cambridge: Cambridge University Press.

COHEN, H. (1953) The evolution of the concept of disease. *Proceedings of the Royal Society of Medicine*, **48**, 155–160.

COHEN, J. (1960) A coefficient of agreement for nominal scales. *Educational and Psychological Measurement*, **20**, 37–46.

COHEN, J. (1968) Weighted kappa: nominal scale agreement with provision for scaled disagreement or partial credit. *Psychological Bulletin*, **70**, 213–220.

COOPER, J. E., KENDELL, R. E., GURLAND, B. J., SHARPE, L., COPELAND, J. R. M. & SIMON, R. (1972) Psychiatric Diagnosis in New York and London. *Maudsley Monograph* No. 20, London: Oxford University Press.

COPELAND, J. R. M., COOPER, J. E., KENDELL, R. E. & GOURLAY, A. J. (1971) Differences in usage of diagnostic labels amongst psychiatrists in the British Isles. *British Journal of Psychiatry*, **118**, 629–640.

COWIE, V. (1961) The incidence of neurosis in the children of psychotics. *Acta Psychiatrica Scandinavica*, **37**, 37–87.

CROOKS, J., MURRAY, I. P. C. & WAYNE, E. J. (1959) Statistical methods applied to the clinical diagnosis of thyrotoxicosis. *Quarterly Journal of Medicine*, **28**, 211–234.

DAVIS, H. (1974) What does the P scale measure? *British Journal of Psychiatry*, **125**, 161–167.

ELSTEIN, A. S., KAGAN, N., SHULMAN, L. S., HILLIARD, J. & LOUPE, M. J. (1972) Methods and theory in the study of medical inquiry. *Journal of Medical Education*, **47**, 85–92.

ENDICOTT, J. & SPITZER, R. L. (1972) Current and Past Psychopathology Scales (CAPPS): rationale, reliability and validity. *Archives of General Psychiatry*, **27**, 678–687.

ENGELSMANN, F., VINAR, O., PICHOT, P., HIPPIUS, H., GIBERTI, F., ROSSI, L. & OVERALL, J. (1970) International comparison of diagnostic patterns. *Transcultural Psychiatric Research*, **7**, 130–137.

ENGLE, R. L. (1963) Medical diagnosis: past, present and future. II Philosophical foundations and historical development of our concepts of health, disease and diagnosis. *Archives of Internal Medicine*, **112**, 520–529.

ESSEN–MÖLLER, E. (1961) On classification of mental disorders. *Acta Psychiatrica Scandinavica*, **37**, 119–126.

ESSEN–MÖLLER, E. (1971) Suggestions for further improvement of the international classification of mental disorders. *Psychological Medicine*, **1**, 308–311.

ESSEN–MÖLLER, E. (1973) Standard lists for threefold classification of mental disorders. *Acta Psychiatrica Scandinavica*, **49**, 198–212.

ESSEN–MÖLLER, E. & WOHLFAHRT, S. (1947) Suggestions for the amendment of the official Swedish classification of mental disorders. *Acta Psychiatrica et Neurologica Scandinavica*, Suppl. **47**, 551–555.

EVERITT, B. S. (1974) *Cluster Analysis*. London: Heinemann.

EVERITT, B. S., GOURLAY, A. J. & KENDELL, R. E. (1971) An attempt at validation of traditional psychiatric syndromes by cluster analysis. *British Journal of Psychiatry*, **119**, 399–412.

EWALT, J. R. (1972) Differing concepts of diagnosis as a problem in classification. *American Journal of Psychiatry*, May Suppl. **128**, 18–20.

EYSENCK, H. J. (1950) Criterion analysis: an application of the hypotheticodeductive method to factor analysis. *Psychological Review*, **57**, 38–53.

EYSENCK, H. J. (1951) Schizothymia – cyclothymia as a dimension of personality. *Journal of Personality*, **20**, 345–384.

EYSENCK, H. J. (1955) Psychiatric diagnosis as a psychological and statistical problem. *Psychological Reports*, **1**, 3–17.

EYSENCK, H. J. (1960) Classification and the problem of diagnosis. In *Handbook of Abnormal Psychology*, 1st edn. ed. Eysenck, H. J. pp. 1–31. London: Pitman.

EYSENCK, H. J. (1970) A dimensional system of psychodiagnostics. In *New Approaches to Personality Classification*, ed. Mahrer, A. R. pp. 169–207. New York: Columbia University Press.

EYSENCK, S. B. G. (1956) Neurosis and psychosis: an experimental analysis. *Journal of Mental Science*, **102**, 517–529.

EYSENCK, S. B. G. & EYSENCK, H. J. (1970) Crime and personality: an empirical study of the three-factor theory. *British Journal of Criminology*, **10**, 225–239.

FEIGHNER, J. P., ROBINS, E., GUZE, S. B., WOODRUFF, R. A., WINOKUR, G. & MUNOZ, R. (1972) Diagnostic criteria for use in psychiatric research. *Archives of General Psychiatry*, **26**, 57–63.

FEINSTEIN, A. R. (1964) Scientific methodology in clinical medicine. II Classification of human disease by clinical behaviour. *Annals of Internal Medicine*, **61**, 757–781.

FEINSTEIN, A. R. (1969) Taxonomy and logic in clinical data. *Annals of the New York Academy of Sciences*, **161**, 450–459.

FISHER, R. A. (1936) The use of multiple measurements in taxonomic problems. *Annals of Eugenics*, **7**, 179–184.

FLEISS, J. L. (1972) Classification of the depressive disorders by numerical typology. *Journal of Psychiatric Research*, **9**, 141–153.

FLEISS, J. L., SPITZER, R. L., COHEN, J. & ENDICOTT, J. (1972) Three computer diagnosis methods compared. *Archives of General Psychiatry*, **27**, 643–649.

FLETCHER, C. M., JONES, N. L., BURROWS, B. & NIDEN, A. H. (1964) American emphysema and British bronchitis: a standardised comparative study. *American Review of Respiratory Disease*, **90**, 1–13.

FORGY, E. W. (1968) Discussant's remarks. In *Classification in Psychiatry and Psychopathology*, eds. Katz, M. M., Cole, J. O. & Barton, W. E. pp. 410–415. Washington, DC: *Public Health Service Publication* No. 1584.

FOULDS, G. A. (1955) The reliability of psychiatric and the validity of psychological diagnoses. *Journal of Mental Science*, **101**, 851–862.

FOULDS, G. A. (1965) *Personality and Personal Illness*. London: Tavistock Publications.

FOULDS, G. A. (1973) The relationship between the depressive illnesses. *British Journal of Psychiatry*, **122**, 531–533.

FRANK, G. H. (1969) Psychiatric diagnosis: a review of research. *Journal of General Psychology*, **81**, 157–176.

FREUDENBERG, R. K. & ROBERTSON, J. P. S. (1956) Symptoms in relation to psychiatric diagnosis and treatment. *Archives of Neurology and Psychiatry*, **76**, 14–22.

GARMEZY, N. (1968) Process and reactive schizophrenia: some conceptions and issues. In *Classification in Psychiatry and Psychopathology*. eds. Katz, M. M., Cole, J. O., & Barton, W. E. pp. 419–466. Washington DC: *Public Health Service Publication* No. 1584.

GAURON, E. F. & DICKINSON, J. K. (1966a). Diagnostic decision making in psychiatry. I. Information usage. *Archives of General Psychiatry*, **14**, 225–232.

GAURON, E. F. & DICKINSON, J. K. (1966b) Diagnostic decision making in psychiatry. II. Diagnostic styles. *Archives of General Psychiatry*, **14**, 233–237.

GAURON, E. F. & DICKINSON, J. K. (1969) The influence of seeing the patient first on diagnostic decision making in psychiatry. *American Journal of Psychiatry*, **126**, 199–205.

GENERAL REGISTER OFFICE (1968) *A Glossary of Mental Disorders. Studies on Medical and Population Subjects* No. 22, London: HMSO.

GOLDBERG, D. P. (1972) The Detection of Psychiatric Illness by Questionnaire. *Maudsley Monograph* No. 21, London: Oxford University Press.

GOLDFARB, A. (1959) Reliability of diagnostic judgements by psychologists. *Journal of Clinical Psychology*, **15**, 392–396.

GRUENBERG, E. M. (1969) How can the new diagnostic manual help? *International Journal of Psychiatry*, **7**, 368–374.

GUILDFORD, J. P. (1954) *Psychometric Methods*, 2nd edn. p. 279. London: McGraw-Hill.

GURNEY, C., ROTH, M., GARSIDE, R. F., KERR, T. A. & SHAPIRA, K. (1972) Studies in the classification of affective disorders. The relationship between anxiety states and depressive illnesses, II. *British Journal of Psychiatry*, **121**, 162–166.

HARDIN, G. (1956) Meaninglessness of the word protoplasm. *Scientific Monthly*, **82**, 112–120.

HEMPEL, C. G. (1961) Introduction to problems of taxonomy. In *Field Studies in the Mental Disorders*, ed. Zubin, J. pp. 3–22. New York: Grune and Stratton.

HEYNS, R. W. & LIPPITT, R. (1954) Systematic observational techniques. In *Handbook of Social Psychology*, ed. Lindzey, G. Vol. **I**, pp. 307–404, Cambridge, Massachusetts: Addison, Wesley.

HOBSON, R. F. (1953) Prognostic factors in electrical convulsive therapy. *Journal of Neurology, Neurosurgery and Psychiatry*, **16**, 275–281.

HOCHE, A. (1910) Die Melancholiefrage. *Zentralblatt für Nervenheilkunde und Psychiatrie*, **21**, 193–203.

HORDERN, A., SANDIFER, M. G., GREEN, L. M. & TIMBURY, G. C. (1968) Psychiatric diagnosis: British and North American concordance on stereotypes of mental illness. *British Journal of Psychiatry*, **114**, 935–944.

HUDGENS, R. W. (1971) The use of the term 'Undiagnosed Psychiatric Disorder'. *British Journal of Psychiatry*, **119**, 529–532.

HUNT, W. A., WITTSON, C. L. & HUNT, E. B. (1953) A theoretical and practical analysis of the diagnostic process. In *Current Problems in Psychiatric Diagnosis*, eds. Hoch, P. H. & Zubin, J. pp. 53–65. New York: Grune and Stratton.

JASPERS, K. (1959) *Allgemeine Psychopathologie*, 7th edn. Translation by Hoenig, J. & Hamilton, M. W. (1962) Manchester: Manchester University Press.

JOHNSON, G., GERSHON, S., BURDOCK, E. I., FLOYD, A. & HEKIMIAN, L. (1971) Comparative effects of lithium and chlorpromazine in the treatment of acute manic states. *British Journal of Psychiatry*, **119**, 267–276.

KANFER, F. H. & SASLOW, G. (1965) Behavioral analysis: an alternative to diagnostic classification. *Archives of General Psychiatry*, **12**, 529–538.

KATZ, M., COLE, J. O. & LOWERY, H. A. (1969) Studies of the diagnostic process: the influence of symptom perception, past experience and ethnic background on diagnostic decisions. *American Journal of Psychiatry*, **125**, 937–947.

KELLY, D. H. W. (1966) Measurement of anxiety by forearm blood flow. *British Journal of Psychiatry*, **112**, 789–798.

KENDELL, R. E. (1968a) The Classification of Depressive Illnesses. *Maudsley Monograph* No. 18, London: Oxford University Press.

KENDELL, R. E. (1968b) An important source of bias affecting ratings made by psychiatrists. *Journal of Psychiatric Research*, **6**, 135–141.

KENDELL, R. E. (1969) The continuum model of depressive illness. *Proceedings of the Royal Society of Medicine*, **62**, 335–339.

KENDELL, R. E. (1973a) Psychiatric diagnoses: a study of how they are made. *British Journal of Psychiatry*, **122**, 437–445.

KENDELL, R. E. (1973b) The influence of the 1968 glossary on the diagnoses of English psychiatrists. *British Journal of Psychiatry*, **123**, 527–530.

KENDELL, R. E., COOPER, J. E., GOURLAY, A. J., COPELAND, J. R. M., SHARPE, L. & GURLAND, B. J. (1971) Diagnostic criteria of American and British psychiatrists. *Archives of General Psychiatry*, **25**, 123–130.

KENDELL, R. E., EVERITT, B., COOPER, J. E., SARTORIUS, N. & DAVID, M. E. (1968) The reliability of the 'Present State Examination'. *Social Psychiatry*, **3**, 123–129.

KENDELL, R. E. & GOURLAY, J. (1970a) The clinical distinction between psychotic and neurotic depression. *British Journal of Psychiatry*, **117**, 257–260.

KENDELL, R. E. & GOURLAY, J. (1970b) The clinical distinction between the affective psychoses and schizophrenia. *British Journal of Psychiatry*, **117**, 261–266.

KENDELL, R. E., PICHOT, P. & von CRANACH, M. (1974) Diagnostic criteria of English, French and German psychiatrists. *Psychological Medicine*, **4**, 187–195.

KENDELL, R. E. & POST, F. (1973) Depressive illnesses in late life. *British Journal of Psychiatry*, **122**, 615–617.

KING, G. F. (1954) Research with neuropsychiatric samples. *Journal of Psychology*, **38**, 383–387.

KLINE, N. S., TENNEY, A. M., NICOLAOU, G. T. & MALZBERG, B. (1953) The selection of psychiatric patients for research. *American Journal of Psychiatry*, **110**, 179–185.

KOSTLAN, A. (1954) A method for the empirical study of psychodiagnostics. *Journal of Consulting Psychology*, **18**, 83–88.

KRAMER, M. (1961) Some problems for international research suggested by observations on differences in first admission rates to the mental hospitals of England and Wales and of the United States. In *Proceedings of the Third World Congress of Psychiatry*, Vol. 3. pp. 153–160. Montreal: Toronto University Press.

KRAÜPL TAYLOR, F. (1971) A logical analysis of the medico-psychological concept of disease. *Psychological Medicine*, **1**, 356–364 & **2**, 7–16.

KREITMAN, N. (1961) The reliability of psychiatric diagnosis. *Journal of Mental Science*, **107**, 876–886.

KREITMAN, N., SAINSBURY, P., MORRISSEY, J., TOWERS, J. & SCRIVENER, J. (1961) The reliability of psychiatric assessment: an analysis. *Journal of Mental Science*, **107**, 887–908.

KUBIE, L. S. (1971) Multiple fallacies in the concept of schizophrenia. In *Problems of Psychosis*, ed. Doucet, P. & Laurin, C. pp. 301–311. Amsterdam: Excerpta Medica.

LAWLEY, D. N. & MAXWELL, A. E. (1971) *Factor Analysis as a Statistical Method*, 2nd edn. London: Butterworths.

LEAPER, D. J., GILL, P. W., STANILAND, J. R., HORROCKS, J. C. & De DOMBAL, F. T. (1973) Clinical diagnostic process: an analysis. *British Medical Journal*, **3**, 569–574.

LEARY, T. & COFFEY, H. S. (1955) Interpersonal diagnosis: some problems of methodology and validation. *Journal of Abnormal and Social Psychology*, **50**, 110–124.

LEDLEY, R. S. & LUSTED, L. B. (1959) Reasoning foundations of medical diagnosis. *Science*, **130**, 9–21.

LEHMANN, H. E. (1968) Discussant's remarks. In *Classification in Psychiatry and Psychopathology*, eds. Katz, M. M., Cole, J. O. & Barton, W. E. pp. 330–344. Washington DC: *Public Health Service Publication* No. 1584.

LEHMANN, H. E. (1971) Epidemiology of depressive disorders. In *Depression in the 70's*, ed. Fieve, R. pp. 21–30. Amsterdam: Excerpta Medica.

LEHMANN, H. E., BAN, T. A. & DONALD, M. (1965) Rating the rater. *Archives of General Psychiatry*, **13**, 67–75.

LEWIS, A. J. (1946) Ageing and senility: a major problem of psychiatry. *Journal of Mental Science*, **92**, 150–170.

LEWIS, A. J. (1953) Health as a social concept. *British Journal of Sociology*, **4**, 109–124.

LIDZ, T., FLECK, S. & CORNELISON, A. R. (1965) *Schizophrenia and the Family*. New York: International Universities Press.

LINDER, R. (1965) Diagnosis: description or prescription? A case study in the psychology of diagnosis. *Perceptual and Motor Skills*, **20**, 1081–1092.

LORR, M. (1966) *Explorations in Typing Psychotics*. Oxford: Pergamon Press.

LORR, M. (1970) A typological conception of the behavior disorders. In *New Approaches to Personality Classification*, ed. Mahrer, A. R. pp. 101–116. New York: Columbia University Press.

LORR, M. & KLETT, C. J. (1967) *Inpatient Multidimensional Psychiatric Scale*. Palo Alto, California: Consulting Psychologists Press.

LUBIN, A. (1950) A note on criterion analysis. *Psychological Review*, **57**, 54–57.

LUBIN, A. (1951) Some contributions to the testing of psychological hypotheses by means of statistical multivariate analysis. Unpublished Ph.D. thesis. University of London.

LYERLY, S. B. (1968) A survey of some empirical clustering procedures. In *Classification in Psychiatry and Psychopathology*, eds. Katz, M. M., Cole, J. O. & Barton, W. E. pp. 353–376. Washington, DC: *Public Health Service Publication*, No. 1584.

McKEON, J. J. (1967) *Hierarchical Cluster Analysis*. George Washington University Biometrics Laboratory.

McPHERSON, F. M., PRESLY, A. S., ARMSTRONG, J. & CURTIS, R. H. (1974) 'Psychoticism' and psychotic illness. *British Journal of Psychiatry*, **125**, 152–160.

MASSERMAN, J. H. & CARMICHAEL, H. T. (1938) Diagnosis and prognosis in psychiatry. *Journal of Mental Science*, **84**, 893–946.

MAXWELL, A. E. (1961) Canonical variate analysis when the variables are dichotomous. *Educational and Psychological Measurement*, **21**, 259–272.

MAXWELL, A. E. (1971) Multivariate statistical methods and classification problems. *British Journal of Psychiatry*, **119**, 121–127.

MAXWELL, A. E. (1972) Difficulties in a dimensional description of symptomatology. *British Journal of Psychiatry*, **121**, 19–26.

MAY, J. V. (1922) *Mental Diseases*. p. 246. Boston: R. G. Badger.

MEDICAL RESEARCH COUNCIL CLINICAL PSYCHIATRY COMMITTEE. (1965) Clinical trial of the treatment of depressive illness. *British Medical Journal*, **1**, 881–886.

MEEHL, P. E. (1967) Theory testing in psychology and physics: a methodological paradox. *Philosophy of Science*, **34**, 103–115.

MEHLMAN, B. (1952) The reliability of psychiatric diagnoses. *Journal of Abnormal and Social Psychology*, **47**, 577–578.

MELLOR, C. S. (1970) First rank symptoms of schizophrenia *British Journal of Psychiatry*, **117**, 15–23.

MELROSE, J. P., STROEBEL, C. F. & GLUECK, B. C. (1970). Diagnosis of psychopathology using stepwise multiple discriminant analysis. *Comprehensive Psychiatry*, **11**, 43–50.

MENDLEWICZ, J., FLEISS, J. L. & FIEVE, R. R. (1972) Evidence for X-linkage in the transmission of manic-depressive illness. *Journal of the American Medical Association*, **222**, 1624–1627.

MENNINGER, K. (1948) Changing concepts of disease. *Annals of Internal Medicine*, **29**, 318–325.

MENNINGER, K. (1963) *The Vital Balance: the life process in mental health and illness*. New York: Viking Press.

MEYER, A. (1907) Fundamental conceptions of dementia praecox. *Journal of Nervous and Mental Disease*, **34**, 331–336.

MINER, G. D. (1973) The evidence for genetic components in the neuroses. *Archives of General Psychiatry*, **29**, 111–118.

MORAN, P. A. P. (1966) The establishment of a psychiatric syndrome. *British Journal of Psychiatry*, **112**, 1165–1171.

NATHAN, P. E., GOULD, C. F., ZARE, N. C. & ROTH, M. (1969) A systems analytic model of diagnosis: improved diagnostic validity from median data. *Journal of Clinical Psychology*, **25**, 370–375.

NISWANDER, G. D., HASLERUD, G. M. & WEINSTEIN, A. G. (1966) A reliability study of psychiatric diagnoses. *Diseases of the Nervous System*, **27**, 111–115.

NORRIS, V. (1959) Mental Illness in London. *Maudsley Monograph* No. 6, London: Chapman and Hall.

NYSTROM, S. (1965) On relation between clinical factors and efficiency of E.C.T. in depression. *Acta Psychiatrica Scandinavica*, Suppl. 181.

OLDHAM, P. D., PICKERING, G., FRASER ROBERTS, J. A. & SOWRY, G. S. C. (1960) The nature of essential hypertension. *Lancet*, **1**, 1085–1093.

OTTOSSON, J. O. & PERRIS, C. (1973) Multidimensional classification of mental disorders. *Psychological Medicine*, **3**, 238–243.

OVERALL, J. E. (1971) Major phenomenological sub-types in a general psychiatric population. *Diseases of the Nervous System*, **32**, 383–387.

OVERALL, J. E. & GORHAM, D. R. (1962) The Brief Psychiatric Rating Scale *Psychological Reports*, **10**, 799–812.

OVERALL, J. E. & GORHAM, D. R. (1963) A pattern probability model for the classification of psychiatric patients. *Behavioral Science*, **8**, 108–116.

OVERALL, J. E., HENRY, B. W. & MARKETT, J. R. (1972) Validity of an empirically derived phenomenological typology. *Journal of Psychiatric Research*, **9**, 87–99.

OVERALL, J. E. & HOLLISTER, L. E. (1964) Computer procedures for psychiatric classification. *Journal of the American Medical Association*, **187**, 583–588.

PASAMANICK, B. (1963) On the neglect of diagnosis. *American Journal of Orthopsychiatry*, **33**, 397–398.

PASAMANICK, B., DINITZ, S. & LEFTON, M. (1959) Psychiatric orientation and its relation to diagnosis and treatment in a mental hospital. *American Journal of Psychiatry*, **116**, 127–132.

PAYKEL, E. S. (1971) Classification of depressed patients: a cluster analysis derived grouping. *British Journal of Psychiatry*, **118**, 275–288.

PAYKEL, E. S. (1972) Depressive typologies and response to amitriptyline. *British Journal of Psychiatry*, **120**, 147–156.

PICHOT, P., BAILLY, R. & OVERALL, J. E. (1966) Les stéréotypes diagnostiques des psychoses chez les psychiatres Français. Comparison avec les stéréotypes Americains. *Proceedings of the Vth International Congress of the Collegium Internationale Neuropsychopharmacologicum.* pp. 16–26. *Excerpta Medica International Congress Series* No. 129.

PILOWSKY, I., LEVINE, S. & BOULTON, D. M. (1969) The classification of depression by numerical taxonomy. *British Journal of Psychiatry*, **115**, 937–945.

POST, F. (1972) The management and nature of depressive illnesses in late life: a follow-through study. *British Journal of Psychiatry*, **121**, 393–404.

PRESLY, A. S. & WALTON, H. J. (1973) Dimensions of abnormal personality. *British Journal of Psychiatry*, **122**, 269–276.

PRIEN, R. F., CAFFEY, E. M. & KLETT, C. J. (1972) A comparison of lithium carbonate and chlorpromazine in the treatment of excited schizo-affectives. *Archives of General Psychiatry*, **27**, 182–189.

PRUSOFF, B. & KLERMAN, G. L. (1974) Differentiating depressed from anxious neurotic out-patients: use of discriminant function analysis for separation of neurotic affective states. *Archives of General Psychiatry*, **30**, 302–309.

RAO, C. R. (1948) The utilisation of multiple measurements in problems of biological classification. *Journal of the Royal Statistical Society (Series B)*, **10**, 159–193.

RAO, C. R. (1968) Discrimination among groups and assigning new individuals. In *Classification in Psychiatry and Psychopathology*, eds. Katz, M. M., Cole, J. O. & Barton, W. E. pp. 229–240. Washington, DC: *Public Health Service Publication* No. 1584.

RAO, C. R. & SLATER, P. (1949) Multivariate analysis applied to differences between neurotic groups. *British Journal of Psychology* (Statistical Section), **2**, 17–29.

RAWNSLEY, K. (1967) An international diagnostic exercise. In *Proceedings of the Fourth World Congress of Psychiatry*. Vol. 4. pp. 2683–2686. Amsterdam: Excerpta Medica Foundation.

REGISTRAR–GENERAL (1856) *Sixteenth Annual Report of the Registrar General of Births, Deaths and Marriages in England*, Appendix, p. 75. London: Eyre and Spottiswoode.

REICH, T., CLAYTON, P. J. & WINOKUR, G. (1969) The genetics of mania. *American Journal of Psychiatry*, **125**, 1358–1368.

REID, J. R. & FINESINGER, J. E. (1952) The role of definitions in psychiatry. *American Journal of Psychiatry*, **109**, 413–420.

RIESE, W. (1953) *The Conception of Disease: its history, its versions and its nature.* New York: Philosophical Library.

ROBERTS, J. M. (1959) Prognostic factors in the electroshock treatment of depressive states. *Journal of Mental Science*, **105**, 703–713.

ROBINS, E. & GUZE, S. B. (1970) Establishment of diagnostic validity in psychiatric illness: its application to schizophrenia. *American Journal of Psychiatry*, **126**, 983–987.

ROSENHAN, D. L. (1973) On being sane in insane places. *Science*, **179**, 250–258.

ROSENZWEIG, N., VANDENBERG, S. G., MOORE, K. & DUKAY, A. (1961) A study of the reliability of the mental status examination. *American Journal of Psychiatry*, **117**, 1102–1108.

RUTTER, M., LEBOVICI, S., EISENBERG, L., SNEZNEVSKIJ, A. V., SADOUN, R., BROOKE, E. & LIN, T. (1969) A triaxial classification of mental disorders in childhood. *Journal of Child Psychology and Psychiatry*, **10**, 41–61.

RUTTER, M., SHAFFER, D. & SHEPHERD, M. (1973) An evaluation of the proposal for a multi-axial classification of child psychiatric disorders. *Psychological Medicine*, **3**, 244–250.

SAGHIR, M. T. (1971) A comparison of some aspects of structured and unstructured psychiatric interviews. *American Journal of Psychiatry*, **128**, 180–184.

SANDIFER, M. G., HORDERN, A. & GREEN, L. M. (1970) The psychiatric interview: the impact of the first three minutes. *American Journal of Psychiatry*, **126**, 968–973.

SANDIFER, M. G., HORDERN, A., TIMBURY, G. C. & GREEN, L. M. (1968) Psychiatric diagnosis: a comparative study in North Carolina, London and Glasgow. *British Journal of Psychiatry*, **114**, 1–9.

SANDIFER, M. G., PETTUS, C. & QUADE, D. (1964) A study of psychiatric diagnosis. *Journal of Nervous and Mental Disease*, **139**, 350–356.

SCADDING, J. G. (1963) Meaning of diagnostic terms in broncho-pulmonary disease. *British Medical Journal*, **2,** 1425–1430.

SCADDING, J. G. (1967) Diagnosis: the clinician and the computer. *Lancet*, **2,** 877–882.

SCADDING, J. G. (1972) The semantics of medical diagnosis. *Biomedical Computing*, **3,** 83–90.

SCHEFF, T. J. (1963) The role of the mentally ill and the dynamics of mental disorder: a research framework. *Sociometry*, **26,** 436–453.

SCHMIDT, H. O. & FONDA, C. P. (1956) The reliability of psychiatric diagnosis: a new look. *Journal of Abnormal and Social Psychology*, **52,** 262–267.

SCHNEIDER, K. (1950) *Die Psychopathischen Persönlichkeiten*. Translation of the 9th edn. by Hamilton, M. W. (1958) pp. 7–10. London: Cassel & Co.

SCHNEIDER, K. (1959) *Klinische Psychopathologie*. Translation of the 5th edn. by Hamilton, M. W. New York: Grune and Stratton.

SEGUIN, C. A. (1946) The concept of disease. *Psychosomatic Medicine*, **8,** 252–257.

SHARPE, L., GURLAND, B. J., FLEISS, J. L., KENDELL, R. E., COOPER, J. E. & COPELAND, J. R. M. (1974) Some comparisons of American, Canadian and British psychiatrists in their diagnostic concepts. *Canadian Psychiatric Association Journal* **19,** 235–245.

SHEPHERD, M., BROOKE, E. M., COOPER, J. E. & LIN, T. (1968) An experimental approach to psychiatric diagnosis. *Acta Psychiatrica Scandinavica*, Suppl. 201.

SHIELDS, J. & GOTTESMAN, I. I. (1973) Cross-national diagnosis of schizophrenia in twins: the heritability and specificity of schizophrenia. *Archives of General Psychiatry*, **27,** 725–730.

SILBERMANN, R. M. (1971) *CHAM: a classification of psychiatric states*. Amsterdam: Excerpta Medica.

SIMON, R. J., GURLAND, B. J., FLEISS, J. L. & SHARPE, L. (1971) Impact of a patient history interview on psychiatric diagnosis. *Archives of General Psychiatry*, **24,** 437–440.

SLATER, E. T. O. (1935) The incidence of mental disorder. *Annals of Eugenics*, **6,** 172–184.

SLETTEN, I. W., ALTMAN, H. & ULETT, G. A. (1971) Routine diagnosis by computer. *American Journal of Psychiatry*, **127,** 1147–1152.

SLETTEN, I. W., ULETT, G., ALTMAN, H. & SUNDERLAND, D. (1970) The Missouri Standard System of Psychiatry. *Archives of General Psychiatry*, **23,** 73–79.

SMITH, W. G. (1966) A model for psychiatric diagnosis. *Archives of General Psychiatry*, **14,** 521–529.

SNEATH, P. H. A. (1957) Some thoughts on bacterial classification. *Journal of General Microbiology*, **17,** 184–200.

SPITZER, R. L., COHEN, J., FLEISS, J. L. & ENDICOTT, J. (1967) Quantification of agreement in psychiatric diagnosis. *Archives of General Psychiatry*, **17,** 83–87.

SPITZER, R. L. & ENDICOTT, J. (1968) Diagno: a computer program for psychiatric diagnosis utilising the differential diagnostic procedure. *Archives of General Psychiatry*, **18,** 746–756.

SPITZER, R. L. & ENDICOTT, J. (1969) Diagno II: further developments in a computer program for psychiatric diagnosis. *American Journal of Psychiatry*, **125,** (Jan. Suppl.), 12–20.

SPITZER, R. L., ENDICOTT, J. & FLEISS, J. L. (1967) Instruments and recording forms for evaluating psychiatric status and history: rationale, method of development and description. *Comprehensive Psychiatry*, **8,** 321–343.

SPITZER, R. L., ENDICOTT, J., FLEISS, J. L. & COHEN, J. (1970) The Psychiatric Status Schedule: a technique for evaluating psychopathology and impairment in role functioning. *Archives of General Psychiatry*, **23,** 41–55.

SROLE, L., LANGNER, T. S., MICHAEL, S. T., OPLER, M. K. & RENNIE, T. A. C. (1962) *Mental Health in the Metropolis: the Midtown Manhattan Study*. New York: McGraw-Hill.

STENGEL, E. (1959) Classification of mental disorders. *Bulletin of the World Health Organization*, **21,** 601–663.

STOER, L. (1964) Agreement between psychiatric and psychological diagnoses in a state hospital. *Journal of Projective Techniques and Personality Assessment*, **28,** 233–240.

STRAUSS, J. S. (1973) Diagnostic models and the nature of psychiatric disorder. *Archives of General Psychiatry*, **29,** 445–449.

STRAUSS, J. S., BARTKO, J. J. & CARPENTER, W. T. (1973) The use of clustering techniques for the classification of psychiatric patients. *British Journal of Psychiatry*, **122,** 531–540.

SZASZ, T. S. (1960) The myth of mental illness. *American Psychologist*, **15,** 113–118.

TAYLOR, J. A. (1953) A personality scale of manifest anxiety. *Journal of Abnormal and Social Psychology*, **48**, 285–295.

TEMERLIN, M. K. (1968) Suggestion effects in psychiatric diagnosis. *Journal of Nervous and Mental Disease*, **147**, 349–353.

THORNDIKE, E. L. (1920) A constant error in psychological ratings. *Journal of Applied Psychology*, **4**, 25–29.

TORGERSON, W. S. (1968) Multidimensional representation of similarity structures. In *Classification in Psychiatry and Psychopathology*, eds. Katz, M. M., Cole, J. O. & Barton, W. E. pp. 212–220. Washington DC: *Public Health Service Publication* No. 1584.

TUKE, H. (1890) French retrospect. *Journal of Mental Science*, **36**, 117–122.

TUKE, H. (1892) *Dictionary of Psychological Medicine*, Vol. 1. London: J. & A. Churchill.

VERMA, R. M. & EYSENCK, H. J. (1973) Severity and type of psychotic illness as a function of personality. *British Journal of Psychiatry*, **122**, 573–585.

WARD, C. H., BECK, A. T., MENDELSON, M., MOCK, J. E. & ERBAUGH, J. K. (1962) The psychiatric nomenclature. *Archives of General Psychiatry*, **7**, 198–205.

WILSON, M. S. & MEYER, E. (1962) Diagnostic consistency in a psychiatric liaison service. *American Journal of Psychiatry*, **119**, 207–209.

WING, J. K., BIRLEY, J. L. T., COOPER, J. E., GRAHAM, P. & ISAACS, A. D. (1967) Reliability of a procedure for measuring and classifying 'Present Psychiatric State'. *British Journal of Psychiatry*, **113**, 499–515.

WING, J. K., COOPER, J. E. & SARTORIUS, N. (1974) *Description and Classification of Psychiatric Symptoms*. Cambridge: Cambridge University Press.

WING, L. (1970) Observations on the psychiatric section of the international classification of diseases and the British glossary of mental disorders. *Psychological Medicine*, **1**, 79–85.

WITTENBORN, J. R., HOLZBERG, J. D. & SIMON, B. (1953) Symptom correlates for descriptive diagnosis. *Genetic Psychology Monographs*, **47**, 237–301.

WOLFE, J. H. (1970) Pattern clustering by multivariate analysis. *Multivariate Behavioural Research*, **5**, 329–350.

WORLD HEALTH ORGANISATION (1948) *Manual of the International Statistical Classification of Diseases, Injuries, and Causes of Death* (ICD–6), *Bulletin of the World Health Organization*, Suppl. 1, Geneva: WHO.

WORLD HEALTH ORGANIZATION (1967) *Manual of the International Statistical Classification of Diseases, Injuries and Causes of Death* (ICD–8), Geneva: WHO.

WORLD HEALTH ORGANIZATION (1973a) *Report of the International Pilot Study of Schizophrenia*. Vol. 1. Geneva: WHO.

WORLD HEALTH ORGANIZATION (1973b) *Report of the Eighth Seminar on Standardisation of Psychiatric Diagnosis, Classification and Statistics*. Geneva: WHO (offset).

ZIGLER, E. & PHILLIPS, L. (1961) Psychiatric diagnosis: a critique. *Journal of Abnormal and Social Psychology*, **63**, 607–618.

ZILBOORG, G. (1941) *A History of Medical Psychology*, New York: W. W. Norton & Co.

ZUBIN, J. (1938) Socio-biological types and methods for their isolation. *Psychiatry*, **1**, 237–247.

ZUBIN, J. (1967) Classification of the behaviour disorders. *Annual Review of Psychology*, **18**, 373–406.

ZUBIN, J. (1968) Biometric assessment of mental patients. In *Classification in Psychiatry and Psychopathology*, eds. Katz, M. M., Cole, J. O. & Barton, W. E. pp. 353–376. Washington, DC: *Public Health Service Publication* No. 1584.

ZUNG, W. K. (1965) A self-rating depression scale. *Archives of General Psychiatry*, **12**, 63–70.

# Author Index

# Subject Index